DEVELOPMENTAL PSYCHOLOGY

Published by
Saurabh Publishing House

DEVELOPMENTAL PSYCHOLOGY

Prof. Padma Sahoo

Saurabh
Publishing House
4735/22, Prakash Deep Building,
Ansari Road, Darya Ganj,
New Delhi - 110002

Published by:

SAURABH PUBLISHING HOUSE

Distributed by:

LOTUS PRESS PUBLISHERS & DISTRIBUTORS
Unit No. 220, Second Floor, 4735/22, Prakash Deep Building,
Ansari Road, Darya Ganj, New Delhi - 110002
Ph: 32903912, 23280047 • E-mail: lotus_press@sify.com

Saurabh Publishing is an imprint of
Lotus Press

Developmental Psychology

ISBN : 978-81-89005-91-7 (H/B)

Printed in India by Concept Imprint, Delhi

Preface

Development describes the growth of humans throughout the lifespan, from conception to death. The scientific study of human development seeks to understand and explain how and why people change throughout life. This includes all aspects of human growth, including physical, emotional, intellectual, social, perceptual, and personality development.

The scientific study of development is important not only to psychology, but also to sociology, education, and health care. Development does not just involve the biological and physical aspects of growth, but also the cognitive and social aspects associated with development throughout life.

The study of human development is important in a number of subjects, including biology, anthropology, sociology, education, history, and psychology. Most important, however, are the practical applications of studying human development. By better understanding how and why people change and grow, we can then apply this knowledge to helping people live up to their full potential.

There are a number of important issues that have been debated throughout the history of developmental psychology.

The debate over the relative contributions of inheritance and the environment is one of the oldest issues in both philosophy and psychology. Philosophers such as Plato and Descartes supported the idea that some ideas are inborn. On the other hand, thinkers such as John Locke argued for the concept of *tabula rosa*—a belief that the mind is a blank slate at birth, with experience determining our knowledge.

Today, most psychologists believe that it is an interaction between these two forces that causes development. Some aspects of development are distinctly biological, such as puberty. However, the onset of puberty can be affected by environmental factors such as diet and nutrition.

A second important consideration in developmental psychology involves the relative importance of early experiences versus those that occur later in life. Are we more affected by events that occur in early childhood, or do later events play an equally important role?

Psychoanalytic theorists tend to focus upon events that occur in early childhood. According to Freud, much of a child's personality is completely established by the age of five. If this is indeed the case, those who have experienced deprived or abusive childhoods might never adjust or develop normally.

In contrast to this view, researchers have found that the influence of childhood events does not necessarily have a dominating effect over behavior throughout the life. Many people with less-that-perfect childhoods go on to develop normally into well-adjusted adults.

A third major issue in developmental psychology is that of continuity. Does change occur smoothly over time, or through a series of predetermined steps? Some theories of development argue that changes are simply a matter of quantity; children display more of certain skills as they grow older. Other theories outline a series of sequential stages in which skills emerge at certain points of development. This book of Developmental Psychology is for researchers, teachers, Psychologists and for all those associated with development and infant psychology. In preparation of this book I am thankful to my parents, students and to my family for their continues support.

Prof. Padma Sahoo

Contents

1

Developmental Psychology: Nature and Significance

Introduction

There is an underlying propensity for humans to walk due to the operation of an in-built genetic programme applying to all members of the species, being independent of learning, not based upon specific environmental events, and not dependent upon interactions between internal and external factors. It is 'innate', part of 'nature'. There are, on the other hand, a variety of forms of walking to be observed, the variations being due to experiential factors, shoes worn, fitness, load carried, cultural norms and so on, the 'nurture' side of the coin. Thus any given instance of walking can be accounted for by a consideration of the relative contribution of the two sorts of causal factors and their interaction. The same general argument applies to every human ability. It is a model for all development. It is the dominant paradigm.

There are two critical features to the model. First, the two sorts of causes of development are mutually exclusive and exhaustive. That means change is due *either* to innate, internal, genetic, biological factors, *or* to learned, external, environmental ones and between them all possible forms of change are accounted for: they form a dichotomy, the 'nature/nurture' dichotomy. Second, in both cases the structure determining the changes is complete, fully formed, either in the blueprint in the genes which gets 'read out' in development or in the existing structure of the environment which becomes internalized through learning, like the route to work or the company policy on dogs. In both cases it is reformed in the brain, either as the expression of the internal genetic code or as internal representations, 'copies' of the external world. Change based on a preexisting form is called preformation, the second critical feature.

A trip to the moon allowed a natural experiment, a test of the model for the case of walking, but also turns out to pose a challenge to the assumptions underpinning the model in general. The prediction had to be that we expect to find 'odd' walking due to the 'odd' conditions, but it will not be possible to find that this form of locomotion is simply not adopted by a member of the human species generally wanting to get about in no great hurry. And certainly not when the only change to reasonably 'normal' conditions is a reduction in the value of one variable out of the huge number influencing the outcome. The variable in question is gravity. Reduce its value, to one sixth of 'normal', by being on the moon, and what happens the supposedly in-built, genetically fixed, independent-of environment programme fails to operate. The astronauts found that jumping was a more suitable mode of locomotion, for the sort of bodies they had in the sort of conditions they encountered. The prediction that walking would occur and why is based upon the nature/nurture dichotomy, walking in some form being genetically determined. But it didn't happen. It has been suggested that they had practice on earth before they went. They did, but that does not explain how what is supposedly genetically determined failed to occur.

If we can be wrong about something as relatively simple as walking, can we rely upon the validity of the two central assumptions of which it is supposedly just an obvious example, that the 'nature/nurture' dichotomy and causal change by preformation constitute a valid basis for psychological theorizing? If we can't we have a major problem, because every single textbook on development still refers to 'innate' causes, to 'biological' influences, to 'predispositions', and so on, and contrasts these with the alternative forms of cause, 'learning', 'cultural or social factors', etc., independent of genes and dependent upon experience, thus still assuming the validity of the nature/nurture dichotomy and the critical implicit assumption that causes in development are to be allocated to membership of one or other of these exclusive, preformed (not formed in the interaction) categories.

Interactionism without Interactions

The situation is odd because it is not as if developmental psychologists claim to be preformationists, or to believe in dichotomies. Everyone, but everyone claims allegiance to an interactionist banner. We recognize the facile nature of single cause, passive-child, unidirectional explanations. We see the limitations of focusing on end-points in development, stages, and the need to examine the processes of change themselves. We appreciate the pervasive influence of contexts. As a result, we all believe in multiple forms of influence, complex interactive effects and transactional, constructivist change. There can be no dichotomies here as causes of all sorts are presumed to interact with each other. Yet the newest textbooks do still use, without modification, precisely the same categories of thought and assumptions they purport to deride. We still read about genetic blueprints for development even though we know that a complex of structures and conditions and interactions are also essential for the usual developmental outcomes, not just genes. Where is the interactionism here? If I learn to recognize someone or to learn a language, their face and that language were preformed. Where is the interaction here? And as for some causes being a mixture of what is 'innate' and 'learned', we are never told even in the most general terms how molecular biological mechanisms involving genes can 'mix' with learning mechanisms. Thus it is that we have effects that are supposed to be due to interactions, but are also claimed to be due to fixed features, genes, faces, language, whatever. And thus it is that we are supposed to accept that different sorts of causes can and must interact, yet belong to categories which are exclusive from each other. This is what happens in the midst of a paradigm shift, confusion. Hence there is now an urgent need to put in place assumptions which are consistent with notions of dynamic, interactive change, not based upon a static, non-interactive, anti-contextual model which dichotomies and preformation demands. The lack is holding psychology back, as there is no focus on interactions themselves. They are the source of all development and the key to our understanding of the processes of change.

The Dichotomies Remain

Just to get a glimpse of the difficulty, consider this small sample of statements from prominent developmental psychologists. Karmiloff-Smith often refers to the innate capacities of the human mind. Now these are generally taken to be developmentally fixed and independent of the environment, not dependent upon contingent interactions, but it is clear from the book that Karmiloff-Smith knows this not to be true. I am not saying she is wrong, but that it is confusing. The same course is extremely pro-interactionist, yet tells us that 'Information-for-development is stored in the genes'. If it is stored in the genes it is surely preformed and not formed in interactions.

There is a variety of forms of preformationist explanations and of confusing uses of associated terms. Take 'biological'. The Open University Course on Foundations of

Child Development, referred to earlier, tells us that there are 'biologically rooted individual differences' or 'genetic differences between children'. Here 'biological' and 'genetic' have the same connotation. But when we hear that 'there are biological effects on temperament that are not influenced by genetic differences, for example effects of illness', the terms refer to totally different sorts of causal factors as 'biological' is being *contrasted* with 'psychological'. But no explanation of this paradox is offered. Even avowed ecological psychologists (who should be united in their opposition to dichotomous thinking) are not immune to the use of such language: Claes Von Hofsten in Dent-Reed and ZukowGoldring writes, 'though experience is necessary for developing actions, biology has also prepared the child for acquiring such skills'. The use of this sort of terminology by 'interactionists' shows, I believe, the state of flux thinking is in. And you have the difficulty of being expected to accept a new gloss on psychological development whilst still being expected to work within the language of the old assumptions. So long as we continue to use the language of dichotomies we have an extra barrier to the adoption of a new paradigm.

Some have proposed alternative theoretical frameworks, all dynamic systems views, seeing change as the central feature of any theory of knowledge, stability as the emergence of products which inevitably become involved in new interactions and resultant flux; and they are all ecological in emphasizing the role of context as of critical causal significance in those processes. In direct opposition to basing analysis on mutually exclusive and exhaustive categories such as nature/nurture, organism/environment, biology/culture, mind/body, we are exhorted to recognize the systemic nature of interaction and development in which the boundaries between dichotomous categories dissolve.

Resistance to Change

But be clear, these frameworks have, as yet, been accepted by only a minority. It is no surprise. When assumptions have dominated thinking so profoundly and for so long, it is no small matter to give them up. Nor should we do so without care. I do not expect you to release one way of thinking until and unless you are convinced that the alternative is better. My aim is to supply the grounds for that conviction. There are several obstacles. The use of 'mixed' assumptions, as I have suggested, is one, because it clouds all the relevant distinctions. But there are other sorts of impediments. In the first place, to question these basic assumptions about the nature of things is, by definition, improper, because assumptions are assumed. The reaction thus tends to be defensive, usually taking the form that no one holds these assumptions anymore. But if we do not, why are all the textbooks still using them? In any case, every conversation we ever have depends upon assumptions. If I discuss public transport with someone, I will assume the existence of people, of a variety of sorts of vehicles, trains that travel on railway lines, lorries on roads, and so on. Talk, even thought, is not possible without assumptions. The same applies to theories. So it is never a case of whether we make assumptions, but only of which ones we make.

The Traditional View of Psychological Development

The model implies that the unit of analysis is the organism, that causal change is due to genetic or environmental factors or some unspecified interaction of the two, and that genetic causes are effective independently of experience (innate) while environmental factors are dependent only upon it. The complexity that we observe in behaviour is due to complex, genetic blueprints or to complex, mental representations. The regularity, the sameness observed in human behaviour across cultures or other sources of difference, is due to the mechanisms of genetic regulation, while the differences in behaviour which covary with experience are due to environmental regulation, learning, by which internal representations of external structure are built.

The main psychological components of the developing organism are perception, cognition and action, each of which must be clearly distinguished from the other. No complex behaviour is possible without a set of internal representations, the content of cognition, which is the essential link between the outside world and the inside mind. They are the map and the directions without which we could not intelligently traverse the mental topography, the key to complex action or thought. They and only they allow analysis and validation of the ambiguous and deceptive world of appearances, which is all that perception can provide, and enable the complex decisions which our bodies are then directed to make material. They consist in knowledge which is not limited to particular situations, but is abstract, general, disembedded, free from particular contexts. Contexts in which behaviours occur are thus not central to psychological functioning. This one is problematical because there is so much evidence now for the importance of context, for the view that all cognition is situated. But, as I say, we are in the midst of change.

Finally, a host of factors can influence any given developmental outcome but we can take refuge in the (assumed) knowledge that at least these factors have linear effects (more of a relevant independent variable has more of an effect), and are additive (pertinent factors accumulate in their effects). I will need to show why and how these views are implied, but more, I need to demonstrate that they are incorrect, every one of them. But that is only a start. For the aim, as I say, is to help you embrace an alternative.

The Ecological, Dynamic Systems View

This view could hardly be more different. It is based upon the assumption that the unit of analysis is decidedly not the organism, but the single system comprised by organism/

environment; that the structure and functions of the organism can be understood only in relation to its fit with the environment. Adaptive action, on this view, is action coupled to specific situations, to environmental contingencies, and that means that organisms must have up-to-date knowledge of the environment as they act and think, which itself means that cognition cannot be decoupled from perception, or from action, as if it were it would not be sensitive to change. Perception becomes critical to intelligent thinking and action.

The traditional position assumes an initial lack of coupling between organism and environment and thus requires the construction of a map or representations of the outside on the inside so that the mind is coupled to the external world. Complex action thus depends upon complex representations. The ecological position assumes that psychological systems evolved to inform action in the real, complex world (not the conditions of the laboratory) and were tested and thus selected by their results in action. This argument applies to selection over evolutionary time, and over ontogenetic time, learning. It implies that representations are not the prime consideration in considering how action can be explained. Rather than complex representations being the condition of complex action, perceptions, cognitions and actions organized together, interacting in the most effective way, are the condition of complex thought.

Development is then that progressive emergence of new relations between the two main components in the system, organism and the environment, as a result of interactions between them. It follows from this position that the components, whether these be internal to an organism, like genes, or external, like social norms, could never be accorded the status of a necessary and sufficient causal condition because it is only in the interaction of all the factors that behavioural outcomes emerge. But these component factors are a mixture of those that have evolved over evolutionary time, like having arms, knee joints, etc., those that have arisen more recently, like practices which have been regularly used for several generations, even those that happened but 10 seconds ago, like learning someone's name. This implies that every time an act is to be carried out it will be constrained by, informed by changes that have taken place over a continuum of time extensions, phylogenetic, ontogenetic, and many others. Thus, both sorts of factors, those from phylogeny, 'nature' and those from ontogeny, 'nurture', are necessary, but only part of the total causal flux from which every single change ever emerges.

In summary, rather than factors causing development coming from two exclusive categories, all developmental and behavioural outcomes emerge from the causal interactions of both sorts together. No developmental change or behaviour is ever preformed, not in genes, nor in the structure of environments. It always arises from interactions in the developmental system. We can account for the regularity observed in development only in terms of the regularity of interactions comprising the developmental system, and the regularity of these interactions depends only upon the regular co-occurrence of the components which interact. That means that to understand how development occurs we need to identify the components of the interactions and the outcomes.

The adoption of the tenets of dynamic systems views entails that we do not expect gradual, linear or additive characteristics of change. On the contrary, we predict that we will find that causal change is characterized by discontinuities, sudden shifts, not continuous change, by non-linear movements between steady states and large, qualitative changes with little change in input to the developmental system. Such change is non-additive and unpredictable in that pertinent variables may have no effect, or a huge effect, depending upon the stability of the system.

We can only adapt to the structure (dynamic and complex in its ways of change, but structure nevertheless) of the environment and of ourselves in relation to it. It call structure invariance, after Gibson. It refers to any regularity to which it would be useful take account of, or which informs adaptive action of thought. Any aspect of the environment which is structured, and almost everything is, thereby must have some invariant properties. Does language have structure? Does a ladder have structure? Does a snail, a thunderstorm, bath time? They all do, of course. This does not mean they are completely fixed, it means they are not random, so we can utilize the pattern, the predictability, the invariance. If you feel uneasy with the word 'invariance', 'structure' will generally do the same job. We argue, crucially, that invariance is a property of the environment or the organism and is thus a component in interaction, while information is what is gained from invariances only if the organism involved has the relevant internal structures, perceptual, cognitive, to utilize the invariances.

Interactions, then, are the basis of development. But development is a long, gradual process involving multiple changes and interactions. The relative stability we observe implies a systematicity to the process, hence the developmental system: a system of interactions which are functionally related to each other, so that earlier events provide opportunities for interactions from which new events will occur, new interactions, and so on.

Now, we need to add another factor: all systems are composed of sub-systems, they are nested, so that the body, for instance, is made up of the immune system, digestive system, circulatory system, etc., each of which is itself sub-divided, and the total external environment made up of the cosmic system, within that the solar system, the earth system, and more local ecologies and effects. The sub-systems always have to function within the constraints of the general system of which they are apart. All organisms and all their adaptations are constrained by the broader system of physical laws that operate, like gravity. All the physiological sub-systems are designed within the general constraints that organisms are self-promoting, active, exchanging energy with their environment, reproducing, etc. That is, no organism is fixed in its design by those constraints (all organisms would be the same if they were), but none are designed other than within the constraints. The point is that the larger system constrains in a generic way the organization of the sub-systems, while the sub-systems have a more specific function and a more differentiated effect. Hence developmental explanation must take account of the nested hierarchical nature of the organism and its environment and the two together.

Human development consists initially in generic systems of knowledge production, which constrain in a general way the psychological structures which exist, channelling them in certain directions and limiting the sorts of problems the infant has to deal with, and that the solution of such problems gives more differentiated knowledge. Each successive set of solutions affords new problems to be tackled with the ever more powerful and differentiated structures at its disposal. The organism becomes more differentiated, as does the effective environment and as does the coupling between organism and environment.

One example might help a little here. Neonates detect and preferentially attend to the regular use of exaggerated rise and fall of tone of voice (invariances in prosody) used by 'mothers', apparently everywhere, called 'motherese'. The 'motherese' is an undifferentiated, generic form of communication, and its effects are pretty undifferentiated, as they do not specify any specific facts will be learned, but the preferential attention to 'mother' does typically ensure that learning about how prosodic features relates to other aspects of mothers' behaviour, and to the infants' feelings, about how prosodic features co-vary with words, etc. does occur. Preferential attention to 'motherese' constrains learning in that attention is focused on these limited aspects of the world, not on others. The broad system, species-typical in this and many cases, produces relatively undifferentiated information, but it serves to organize what sorts of learning will occur, and this learning is more specific and differentiated. The more generic interactions afford the more specific ones. This is how knowledge develops.

□□□

2

Developmental Psychology and Genetic Change

Introduction

The focus of the field on developmental genetic change lends credence to, and will eventually provide the foundation for, the concept of genetic change as the essence of developmental behavioural genetics. If genetic changes did not occur during development, there would be little use for the field because the behavioural genetic story at any point in development-infancy, childhood, adolescence, adulthood—would be the same elsewhere in the life span. However, developmental change throughout the life span is patently obvious, and it would be incredible if genetic effects were not involved in these changes.

The term genetic change in developmental behavioural genetics really means changes in the effects of genes on behavioural differences among individuals. It is in this sense that developmental behavioural genetics was described as the "bottom line." It ascribes variance in a population to genetic and environmental origins regardless of the molecular mechanisms by which genetic variation among individuals emerges—in developmental behavioural genetics, genetic change is a population concept, not a polypeptide concept. This is fortunate because molecular genetic research has shown that development in eukaryotes is complex, with many possible regulatory mechanisms that seem to work in concert as rheostats rather than as simple on/off switches as in prokaryotes. These facts are likely to combine to snarl the study of genetic mechanisms interwoven in the processes of behavioural development.

Another way in which *genetic change* means something different in developmental behavioural genetics is that it refers to variance in a population. Developmental behavioural genetics does not speak to genetic universals that is, that you and I share many nonvarying stretches of DNA and that we both share a large proportion of these with other primates and other mammals. No doubt some of these nonvarying genes govern developmental changes universal to all mammals and all primates, as well as to our species; molecular geneticists are primarily interested in such genetic phenomena. However, developmental behavioural genetics is limited to the study of genetic effects upon behavioural differences among individuals in a population.

From the perspective of developmental behavioural genetics, genetic change can be viewed in two major ways: as changes in the relative magnitude of genetic and environmental variance for a particular characteristic, and as changes in genetic covariance during development.

Developmental Changes

Heritability is a descriptive statistic referring to the portion of observed variability that can be accounted for by genetic differences among individuals. The rest of the variance, the nongenetic portion, has been called environmentality. Although these descriptive statistics often raise hackles, they are merely a convenient shorthand for describing genetic and environmental components of phenotypic variance. When we say that heritability can change during development, we mean that the relative roles of genetic and environmental influences can change during development in terms of their effects on behavioural differences among individuals in the population. For example, the twin method assesses heritability by examining the magnitude of the difference between correlations for identical twins (who are 100% similar genetically) and those for fraternal twins (who are roughly 50% similar genetically for segregating genes). Thus, a change in heritability means that the difference between identical and fraternal twin correlations changes. If heritability increases during development, the difference in correlations increases because the identical twin correlation increases or the fraternal twin correlation decreases.

It should be clear that developmental changes in heritability do not implicate molecular mechanisms of change. For example, heritability could increase from one age to another even if the same genes were actively transcribed at both ages: If environmental variance declines during development, genetic variance accounts for a relatively larger portion of the phenotypic variance.

Although developmental changes in heritability are not especially informative for molecular geneticists, it could be useful for psychologists to know, for example, that variance for a trait of interest is entirely due to environmental variance early in development and then becomes increasingly affected by genetic variance as development proceeds. Although few developmentalists have considered the issue of developmental change in heritability, most would probably guess the reverse to be closer to the truth: As children develop, they experience more diverse environments and thus environmental variance will increasingly account for phenotypic variance. In other words, heritability will decrease during development. This is explicitly the view among Soviet developmentalists. However, as we shall see in later chapters, when developmental change in heritability is found, it always occurs in the opposite direction: Heritability increases during development.

Early Studies

The earliest studies in human behavioural genetics were focused on this issue. Galton studied the life histories of two groups of twins: those in which twin partners were similar to each other early in development, and those in which the twins were dissimilar. Galton investigated the extent to which the twins' initial similarity or dissimilarity changed during development and concluded that the initial resemblance of twins was maintained throughout life. Galton was primarily interested in testing the influence of environment, reasoning that twins in a family, because they experience more similar environments than do twins in different families, should become more similar if the family environment is important. If the groups of initially similar and initially dissimilar twins were identical and fraternal twins, respectively, Galton's results would suggest that heritability does not change. However, this assumption cannot be made because identical twins are often less similar than fraternal twins early in life for example, identical twins show larger birth weight differences than fraternal twins. If heritability increases during development and if Galton's groups each contained identical and fraternal twins, no changes in twin resemblance would be detected because identical twin correlations would increase and fraternal twin correlations would decrease.

The well-known learning theorist, E.L. Thorndike, conducted a similar study in 1905 using objective measures of specific cognitive abilities. He found that 9 and 10-year-old twins showed the same degree of similarity as 13- and 14-year-old twins. Thorndike did not believe that there were two types of twins and made no attempt to separate the twins in his study. Thus, his sample contained approximately equal numbers of identical and fraternal twins and therefore could not reveal developmental changes in heritability.

Merriman conducted the first methodologically valid twin study comparing identical and fraternal twins for IQ. However, to study developmental change, he divided the entire twin sample into two groups, those 5 to 9 years old and those 10 to 16 years old, regardless of zygosity. As in the studies by Galton and by Thorndike, he found no difference in the IQ correlations for the younger and the older groups.

Because none of these early studies considered changes in the relative magnitude of identical and fraternal twin correlations during development, they do not speak to the issue of developmental change in heritability.

Analyzing Developmental Change in Heritability

Rather than dividing twin samples into younger and older pairs, a far more powerful method for analyzing changes in heritability during development is hierarchical multiple regression. The procedure begins with the regression of one twin partner's score on the other twin partner's score, a measure of twin resemblance. Data on the twins, say identical twins, are entered in double-entry format (each twin's scores are duplicated, the score for twin partner B follows the score for twin A on the "independent variable," and B's data precede A's data for the "dependent variable") in order to equalize means and variances, which makes this regression equivalent to the usual twin intra class correlation. Thus, a significant standardized partial regression coefficient indicates significant twin resemblance. The twins' age is added as a second variable in the multiple regression. Then another variable is constructed to represent the two-way interaction between twin score and age simply by obtaining the product of twin score and age for each individual. The multiple regression is called "hierarchical" because variance due to "main effects" (twin score and age) is removed in a first step before the significance of the interaction term is tested. (This is exactly what is done in the computational short-cut for multiple regression using discrete groups which is known as analysis of variance.) A significant standardized partial regression coefficient for the interaction term implies a conditional relationship: Twin resemblance differs as a function of age. Various procedures can be used to determine the direction of the age changes in twin resemblance, but the simplest is to dichotomize the sample (e.g., most and least similar twins; youngest and oldest twins) and examine the means of the four cells for the dependent measure.

This procedure can be repeated with fraternal twins and the results of the hierarchical multiple regressions for identical and fraternal twins can b6 compared. However, a considerably more efficient and more powerful procedure is to include data from both identical and fraternal twins in a single HMR analysis, adding a third variable, zygosity. Zygosity is a "dummy" variable indicating whether each individual is a member of an identical twin pair or a fraternal pair. The coefficient of relationship (1.0 for identical twins and .50 for fraternal twins) could be used to code zygosity. The significance of each of the three main effects is tested first in the hierarchical analysis. The second step tests the three two-way interactions (twin score age, twin score zygosity, age zygosity). For example, a significant two way interaction between twin score and zygosity implies that twin resemblance differs as a function of zygosity that is, heritability is significant. Of most interest is the three-way interaction (twin score age zygosity) which is tested in the third step. A significant three-way interaction means that heritability (i.e., twin score zygosity) differs as a function of age. If significant interactions are found, additional analyses need to be conducted to determine whether heritability increases or decreases with age.

Table 2.1. Sample Sizes (Twin Pairs) Needed for Detecting Significant Three-Way Interactions (Developmental Change in Heritability Using Twin Data) with 80% Power and p < .05 Using Hierarchical Multiple Regressional

b^2: The Amount Variance Accounted for by the Interaction Effect	**R^2: The Amount of Variance Accounted for by of Main and Interaction Effects Together**							
	.01	**.05**	**.10**	**.20**	**.30**	**.40**	**.50**	**.60**
.01		748	709	628	552	471	395	316
.05			143	128	112	96	81	65
.10				65	57	49	41	33
.20					29	26	22	18

It should be noted that large samples are needed to assess developmental changes in heritability; small samples will not detect such change. Statistical power for detecting a significant three-way interaction depends on the "effect size" the magnitude of the change in heritability during the developmental span under study and also on the overall R^2 of the HMR as well as the sample size. Table 2.1 indicates the sample sizes (number of twin pairs of each type) needed to obtain 80% power to detect a significant three-way interaction (i.e., to detect a significant change in heritability 80% of the time) for reasonable combinations of b^2 (total variance explained by the three-way interaction) and R^2 with $p < .05$. For example, if the HMR yields an R^2 of .50, a three-way interaction accounting for 1% of the total variance (2% of the explained variance) requires a sample size of 395 for 80% power. If the three-way interaction explains 5% of the total variance, a sample size of 81 is needed. This means that over 80 pairs of identical twins and 80 pairs of fraternal twins are needed to detect a change in heritability that accounts for 5% of the variance of twins' scores in an HMR analysis whose overall R^2 is 50%. Despite its need for large sample sizes, HMR is considerably more powerful than arbitrarily dichotomizing samples into younger and older twins; furthermore, from a conceptual point of view, age is a continuous variable and should thus be analyzed in a continuous manner.

The HMR can also be applied to other behavioural genetic designs to explore developmental changes in heritability. For example, because resemblance of identical twins reared apart directly assesses heritability, the two-way interaction between separated identical twins' scores and their age directly assesses heritability as a function of age.

In summary, one way to conceptualize genetic change in development is as a change in heritability, and HMR is a useful procedure for such analyses. Although few studies have systematically examined this issue of genetic change, reviews of research on the major developmental epochs lead to the conclusion that, when heritability changes during development, it increases. Such research is discussed in later chapters. However, changes in heritability do not speak to the issue of the covariation of genetic effects at different points during development that is the topic of the following section.

Genetic Correlations in Development

Developmental change in heritability is essentially a cross-sectional concept. The second concept of genetic change addresses the genetic contribution to longitudinal, age-to-age change and continuity. Age-to-age genetic correlations indicate the extent to which genetic effects at one age correlate with genetic effects at another age. To the extent that genetic variance at two ages does not covary, genetic change is implicated. Identification of genetic sources of developmental change is important because change prevails over continuity for most aspects of development. For this reason, a major task for developmental behavioural genetics is to explain longitudinal change, not just continuity. Developmental transitions such as those seen in cognitive development in the second year, at 5-7 years, and at 11-13 years could be due to genetic reorganization: Age-to age genetic correlations would be expected to dip during transitional periods.

Developmental Genetic Change and Familial Resemblance

A fundamental tenet of genetics is that first-degree relatives share roughly half of their segregating genes. Some qualifications have long been understood. For example, siblings share half of their segregating genes only on the average for a particular sibling pair, it depends on how many chromosomes from their mother and father they happen to have in common. Also, the statement applies only to additive genetic variance; siblings also share one-quarter of nonadditive genetic variance due to dominance. Thus, to the extent that nonadditive genetic effects are important, siblings share more than half of their segregating genes.

Parents and their offspring share only additive genetic variance; however, assortative mating can inflate parent-offspring (and sibling) genetic similarity beyond 50%.

These qualifications of the statement that first-degree relatives share 50% of their segregating genes are well known. However, recognition that genetic effects change during development leads to a new qualification; unless first degree relatives are the same age, we would not expect their effective genetic similarity to be 50%. Twins are exactly the same age and any genetic changes that occur during development will be shared to the extent of their genetic similarity—100% for identical twins and 50% for fraternal twins. However, non twin siblings and, especially, parents and their offspring cannot be expected to display their 50% genetic similarity unless they are studied at the same ages.

Of course, no one would test members of a twin pair at different ages. However, with siblings and, especially, with parents and offspring, it is usually a practical necessity to test family members at different ages. In this case, genetic similarity between the relatives depends on the extent of genetic change during development, as indexed by the genetic correlation.

Amplification Model of Developmental Genetics

In summary, genetic change during development can involve changing heritabilities and genetic correlations less than unity. These components affect expectations for parent-offspring resemblance.

All combinations of changing heritabilities and genetic correlations are possible. The prevailing view among developmentalists that individual differences in infancy are not at all predictive of later variability would lead to Model A: Regardless of the relative heritabilities in infancy and adulthood, no genetic continuity exists. Moderates might go along with Model B, slight genetic overlap between infancy and adulthood, as a possibility. One of the most exciting findings to emerge from the CAP data is support for the surprising Model C, which suggests nearly complete genetic overlap between infancy and adulthood. That is, when genetic influence is found in infancy, it covaries nearly completely with adult genetic variance. Moreover, a substantial increase in genetic variance from infancy to adulthood (the right side of Model C) makes it necessary to posit an amplification model of gene action, as explained in this section.

IQ. To understand these conclusions, it is necessary to bring together the concepts discussed previously in this chapter. Using IQ as an example, the CAP infancy results suggest a correlation of about .10 between biological parents' IQ and adopted-away infants' Bayley Mental Development Index (MDI) scores. Although this correlation is small, our previous discussion of the impact of genetic changes during development on parent-offspring correlations led to the expectation of correlations of this magnitude for reasonable combinations of heritability and genetic correlations. Moreover, maximum-likelihood, model-fitting approaches confirm significant genetic variance when the biological parents' data are analyzed simultaneously with adoptive parents' data and data from non adoptive families. Finally, taken at face value, this implies that 20% of the variance is due to heredity, and it is rare in the behavioural sciences that we can explain 20% of the variance.

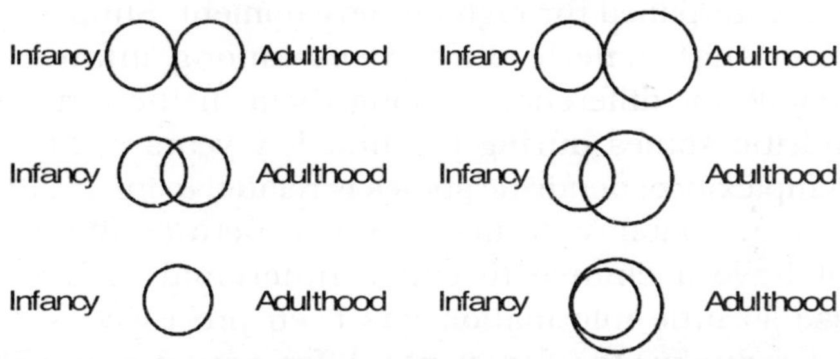

At the simplest level, significant resemblance between biological parents (who are, of course, adults) and their adopted-away infants implies some genetic continuity from infancy to adulthood. We can be more precise. The expected correlation between biological parents and their adopted-away children it is the usual 50% weighted by the heritabilities in childhood and adulthood and the genetic correlation between childhood and adulthood. To estimate the genetic correlation, we need to employ estimates of heritabilities in infancy and adulthood. The heritability of adult IQ is usually taken to be about 50%.

The reason why these estimates of genetic correlation are so high is that heritability in infancy is low. Given significant resemblance between biological parents and their adopted-away infants, this small amount of genetic variance in infancy must covary substantially with genetic variance in adulthood. This is why the right-hand side of

Model C in Figure was selected as best fitting the facts of increasing genetic variance and substantial genetic correlation from infancy to adulthood.

The estimate of genetic correlation for IQ from infancy to adulthood for IQ is so great that it poses a problem: How can the genetic correlation be nearly1.0 when genetic variance increases so substantially from infancy to adulthood? This question is what led DeFries (personal communication) to pose the amplification model of developmental genetics: Genes that affect IQ make only a small contribution to phenotypic variance at first, but their effects are amplified throughout development. Suppose, for example, that genetic differences among infants are responsible for differences among them in the formation of dendritic spines during the first few years of life and that complexity of dendritic spines is related to information-processing capability. At first, these structural differences do not have a chance to cause functional differences because so little information has been processed at that point. Gradually, the functional differences are amplified as more and more information is processed by children. If wc were to measure differences in categorization ability early in childhood, the genetic differences among children due to the complexity of dendritic spines would contribute a negligible amount of variance to observed variability among the children in categorization ability. The differences snowball as development proceeds, so that a study of the children when they are older will show more genetic variance. Yet the genetic correlation between the two ages is near unity because the genetic portion of observed variability at both ages originates with the same set of genes whose effects become amplified during development. In other words, even though genetic variance is relatively less important early in development than it is later, the little genetic variance that does exist in early childhood is substantially related to the genetic variance that affects the trait later in life.

The amplification model makes some strong and testable predictions. For example, it predicts that as the CAP children grow older, the genetic correlations from childhood to adulthood as estimated from parent-offspring correlations will continue to approach unity even though heritability increases. The model also predicts that longitudinal twin data will show a similar pattern of high age-to-age genetic correlations and increasing heritability from infancy to middle childhood. The data from the Louisville Twin Study could provide this information, although they have not as yet been analyzed in terms of age-to-age genetic correlations. It should be noted that the amplification model does not predict high phenotypic correlations from age to age, just high genetic age-to-age correlations. A related prediction from the amplification model is that increasing stability for IQ during childhood comes about because the high age-to-age genetic correlation begins to account for more of the phenotypic variance. That is, heritability increases and the high genetic correlation from age to age shows up in increasing phenotypic stability. This could explain the apparent relationship between heritability and stability in development.

It should be mentioned that the amplification model does not require that the processes underlying the measures be isomorphic in infancy and adulthood. For example, genetic continuity from infant Bayley MDI scores to adult IQ might be due to entirely different processes in infancy and adulthood. "Infancy genes" might affect rate of language acquisition, for example, whereas "adult genes" might affect symbolic reasoning. However, it is also possible that similar cognitive processes are involved at both ages, as has been argued in the case of infant novelty preference. The amplification model apparently is not limited to IQ: The model has been found to apply to physical characteristics as well.

Height and Weight. Data for height and weight are useful as "anchor" points for comparison to behavioural data.

For these traits, a substantial genetic correlation from infancy to adulthood would not be as surprising as it is in the case of IQ because phenotypic stability is apparent for physical characteristics. For height, the correlation between infancy and adulthood is .67 at 12 months and .75 at 24 months; for weight, the correlations are .42 and .48. In the CAP, the correlation between biological mothers and their adopted-away offspring is .32 at both 12 and 24 months, similar to the correlations for nonadoptive parents and their offspring. For weight, the correlations are slightly lower, about .25. These significant correlations between biological mothers and their adopted-away offspring indicate genetic continuity from infancy to adulthood.

The amplification model predicts that as genes come to affect a character in infancy, they will continue to affect the character in adulthood. In other words, genetic covariance between infancy and adulthood accounts for nearly all of the genetic variance in infancy. For height and weight, unlike Bayley MDI scores, heritabilities are substantial in infancy: .70 and .68, respectively. The heritability of height in adulthood is about .90; the heritability of weight is about .80. Combined with the correlations for biological mothers and their adopted-away offspring, these data do, in fact, lead to estimates of substantial genetic correlations.

The genetic correlations of about .80 and .70 for height and weight corroborate the amplification model: Although genetic variance accounts for somewhat less of the phenotypic variance in infancy than in adulthood, the genetic covariance between infancy and adulthood is substantial.

Other Domains. Other domains of development are not nearly as well studied as are IQ and physical characteristics. Although the amplification model might not generalize to all domains of development, some support for the model was found in the CAP data on shyness, which appears to be one of the most heritable dimensions of temperament throughout the life span. At 24 months of age, adoptees' shyness as rated by their adoptive parents correlated significantly with biological mothers' self-reports of sociability. Although the heritabilities of infant shyness or adult sociability are not known precisely, twin studies generally suggest at least moderate heritability in infancy and substantial heritability in adulthood. Assuming a heritability of .30 for infants and .50 for adults, the genetic correlation between infancy and adulthood is .78; if the heritabilities in infancy and adulthood are both .30, the genetic correlation between infancy and adulthood is 1.0. In either case, substantial genetic continuity between infant shyness and adult sociability is predicted.

This example of genetic continuity between infant shyness and adult sociability raises a problem in terms of falsifying the amplification model. If we examine only traits selected because they show significant correlations between biological parents and their adopted-away offspring, we are loading the deck in favour of finding genetic continuity from infancy to adulthood: A significant correlation between biological parents and adopted-away offspring in itself indicates that some genetic continuity must be present. On the other hand, if we examine traits that are completely different in infancy and adulthood (even if they are given the same labels), no parent-offspring resemblance will be found because the genetic correlation from infancy to adulthood is zero. If these traits are found to be heritable in infancy and in adulthood, the results would appear to speak against the amplification model because, in this case, genetic variance in infancy is not found to covary highly with genetic variance in adulthood.

For example, next to shyness, the temperament that shows the best evidence for heritability in infancy from twin studies is emotionality. However, the CAP parent-offspring data yield no evidence for genetic influence. Does this violate the amplification model? If we play the role of devil's advocate, it does. Yet the obvious differences between infant "emotionality" and adult "emotionality" leave some doubt: Measures of infant emotionality assess how often the baby cries and fusses, whereas adult emotionality involves fear and anger.

As a safeguard against studying completely different traits in infancy and adulthood, disconfirmation of the amplification model should involve showing some, but only slight, genetic correlation from infancy to adulthood. Height presented a reasonable opportunity for disconfirming the model. If the correlation between biological parents and their adopted- away offspring had been .10 rather than .32, the genetic correlation from infancy to adulthood would have been .13 rather than .81. Because we already know that height correlates highly within individuals from infancy to adulthood, finding a genetic correlation of .13 between infancy and adulthood would strikingly disconfirm the model.

Even if the amplification model does not generalize to other domains, it is exciting that it does appear to apply to mental development and to height and weight. One implication with practical significance is that heritability of infant scores could be used as a criterion to maximize the prediction of adult scores from scores in infancy.

Summary

The concept of genetic change during development is the theme of this chapter. A cross-sectional look at genetic change involves age-to-age changes in heritability. Longitudinal behavioural genetic data can be used to estimate age-to-age genetic correlations, which index genetic change as well as genetic continuity. The amplification model suggests that as genes come to affect a trait in infancy, they increasingly affect the variance of the trait as their effects are amplified. Although genetic continuity is emphasized in the amplification model, the need for the model arises because of observed genetic change in heritabilities. The possibility that genetic effects become amplified as development proceeds seems the only way to explain high age-to-age genetic correlations coupled with increases in heritability from age to age.

Although the concept of genetic change is the most fundamental issue in developmental behavioural genetics, other important issues have emerged from the application of behavioural genetic concepts and methods to research in developmental psychology.

3

Violence, Philanthropy and Self-Regulation

Introduction

Many more extensive and detailed reviews of recent research, from a variety of perspectives, are available elsewhere. The questions themsclvcs have been of interest to thoughtful people, in one form or another, at least since the days of Plato, and much of the history of Western philosophy can be read as an attempt either to answer or to avoid them.

This chapter presents an approach to conceptualizing both the possibility of, and the actual emergence and development of, altruistic and aggressive behaviour during childhood.

Aggression and Altruism as Intentional Actions

The activities that we call aggressive and altruistic are, by definition, intentional. Consider, for example, some experiences I might have when riding on a crowded bus or other public conveyance. Perhaps I am pushed or shoved by another passenger. Do I call this behaviour aggressive? I may, but only if I believe that it was done *on purpose;* otherwise, I should think that it was merely inadvertent or accidental, not that it was aggressive. Perhaps I drop some packages, and a fellow passenger, a stranger, picks them up for me. Do I call this action altruistic? Possibly I do, but only if I believe that he did so in my interest; if he subsequently asks me for money, I will likely change my interpretation of his behaviour.

In deciding whether a particular behaviour qualifies as an example of aggression or altruism, then, it is not just the topography or physical characteristics of the behaviour that count. To speak of a person as being "aggressive by accident" or "altruistic for selfish purposes" simply doesn't make sense; in these cases, we say instead that a person's behaviour stems from some other motive or cause. Thus, when we say of a person's behaviour that it is altruistic or aggressive, attribution of *intent* is central to what we mean.

For this reason, it is useful to view both aggressive and altruistic behaviour in the broader context of people's efforts to achieve what I term "self-regulation." In my definition of the term, self-regulation involves the successful achievement, through intentional action, of personally selected aims and goals. The aims themselves, and the actions through which they are realized, can be as varied as the people who conceive them and as different as the individuals who carry them out. Whatever is done freely and successfully to fulfil an intention or intentions can, in this sense, be regarded as self-regulated activity. In the usage adopted here, the domain of self-regulation is coterminous with the realm of effective, intentional action.

Inclusion of aggressive and altruistic practices under the rubric of self-regulation is helpful in part because it calls attention to their status not just as *behaviours*, but also as *actions*. Any movement of a person's body, whether intentional or unintentional, can be thought of as behaviour. As I employ the term here, it is only that subset of behaviour that we call intentional which is properly thought of as action. Thus, those movements of my fellow passenger's body that result in my being jostled as we both ride on a bus are behaviours quite apart from the stranger's intentions, or lack of them. They constitute actions, however, only insofar as they are intended. Aggression and altruism are actions, and actions are intentional behaviours.

The idea of intentional action is useful here because it highlights the importance of descriptions that we use, the importance of our interpretations. Actions are intentional, as Anscombe has shown, only under the particular descriptions or interpretations that we make of them. For example, imagine once again that I drop my packages on a crowded bus. This time, let us assume that a man I do not know stoops down to pick them up for me, and that he jostles other passengers in the process. One interpretation is that this man intended to offer me help, and that he accidentally pushed or shoved other people in his attempt to do so. In this case, we might say that his actions were altruistic.

Another interpretation might be that, for whatever reasons of his own (let us say that he was a pickpocket, or that he knew and disliked other passengers on the bus), he intended to jostle other passengers, and simply seized on my fallen parcels as an opportunity to do so. In this case, we might call his actions aggressive. In either case, however, it is our interpretation of his intentions which creates for us the meaning of his action, whether altruistic or aggressive. Seeing aggression and altruism as cases of intentional action helps to highlight the importance of interpretation in their understanding.

One implication of this view is that whether a particular behaviour will be called an aggressive or an altruistic act indeed, whether it will be called an act at all may depend upon the viewpoint of the person who is doing the calling. The man who jostles me on the bus and I myself who am jostled may have very different interpretations of what it is that he was trying or intending to do; hence, the two of us may literally see his single set of movements as different actions. We return to this point later on, when considering research on the development of altruism and aggression in childhood, because there the possibility will emerge that what appears to us, for example, as a child's aggressive action may appear as something quite different to the child who performs it.

I have thus far suggested that aggression and altruism should be viewed as examples of intentional action, and hence that they should be seen in the context of our efforts to achieve self-regulation; and I have emphasized the centrality of interpretation in the understanding of self-regulated action. I turn now to sketch some of the possible implications of these views.

In the context of altruism and aggression, what might some of these implications be? One of them is that we ought to acknowledge a distinction between behaviour that is violent or aversive on the one hand, and aggressive action on the other. An infant's cry can be extremely aversive to others without being aggressive, without arising out of any intention to hurt or to cause pain. A child's motor activities can be violent (i.e., characterized by strong physical force) and can even inadvertently injure others, without being aggressive. Violent and/or aversive behaviour is a generic category, of which aggressive action is a subset.

In a similar vein, it is important to distinguish between behaviour that has positive or beneficial effects on others, and altruistic action, as such. A young infant who smiles engagingly at his or her caretakers is behaving in a prosocial manner, but is unlikely to be doing so for altruistic reasons. A child who uncomplainingly performs his or her household chores is behaving in a prosocial way, but may or may not be doing this out of altruistic motives. Altruistic action is thus a subset of the much larger category of prosocial behaviour.

By offering these conceptual distinctions between antisocial behaviour and aggressive action on the one hand, and between prosocial behaviour and altruistic action on the other I do not mean to suggest that the activity of distinguishing them in practice is always easy. To the contrary, as the examples considered earlier show, these distinctions can be quite difficult to apply in concrete cases. Because these distinctions are so important to our understanding, however, it is essential that even as we acknowledge the practical difficulties involved in making them, we nevertheless persist in our efforts to do so.

There are a number of reasons why these distinctions are important. One reason is that they remind us that altruistic and aggressive intentions can be realized through a wide variety of activities, including but not limited to those that appear, at a surface level, to be either aversive or rewarding. It is by no means clear, for instance, that altruistic aims cannot sometimes best be accomplished through hurtful or painful means (as, for example, when a close friend tells me something that, although painful to hear, is beneficial to my well-being). Similarly, aggressive aims are sometimes accomplished quite effectively through outwardly pleasant means (as, for example, when a cutting remark is delivered as a joke, or with a smile). Keeping in mind the distinction between topography and intention helps to remind us that the actions undertaken to realize our intentions can take many different forms.

Taking the same point from the other side, these distinctions also remind us that behaviour that is antisocial or prosocial in its outward aspect does not necessarily spring from aggressive or altruistic intentions. Thus, what may at first glance appear as aggression in children may in fact have been activities undertaken to achieve quite different intentions. Hence, these distinctions help to guard against the inappropriate projection of our initial interpretations in cases where they may not fit.

Summary

I have argued that the human activities that we term aggressive and altruistic are, by definition, *intentional* in nature. In other words, I have suggested that aggression and altruism are not simply cases of behaviour, but are cases of intentional behaviour, or *action* as well. From this viewpoint, it follows that not every antisocial behaviour can be considered aggressive, nor can every prosocial behaviour be considered altruistic. Only those antisocial (e.g., violent and/or aversive) actions that we believe to have been undertaken with intent to harm another person ought to be considered aggression; only those prosocial (e.g., pleasant and/or beneficial) actions that we believe to have been undertaken with intent to help another person ought to be considered altruistic. Hence, the interpretation of an actor's intentions is crucial to the identification of aggressive or altruistic action. Because the attribution of intentionality is so central to identification of aggression and altruism, and because various observers may interpret an actor's intentions differently, the very existence of either aggression or altruism is often subject to debate and disagreement in particular cases. This is especially likely to be true when the actor whose behaviour we are seeking to interpret is a very young child.

Emergence and Development of Aggressive Action

Consider the following encounter between two 7-year-olds:

Marian is complaining to all that David had squirted her on the pants she has to wear tonight. She says, "I'm gonna do it to him to see how he likes it." She fills a can with water and David runs to the teacher and tells of her threat. The teacher takes the can from Marian. Marian attacks David and pulls his hair very hard. Later, Marian and Elaine go upstairs and into the room where David is seated with a teacher. He throws a book at Marian. The teacher asks Marian to leave. Marian kicks David, then leaves.

The kicking, hair pulling, and book throwing described in this vignette are clearly intentional behaviour; they are clearly actions. Moreover, they are clearly performed with the intent to injure or harm another; they are clearly aggressive actions. If we were to ask either Marian or David why they acted as they did, we would expect them to reply by expressing their dislike of and/or their desire to hurt the other.

Compare these observations made by Piaget of his infant son:

At 6 months, I present Laurent with a matchbox, extending my hand laterally to make an obstacle to his prehension. Laurent tries to pass over my hand, or to the side, but he does not attempt to displace it. These and similar reactions continue essentially unchanged for several weeks. Finally, at 7 months 13 days, Laurent reacts quite differently. I present a box of matches above my hand, but behind it, so that he cannot reach it without setting the obstacle aside. But Laurent, after trying to take no notice of it, suddenly tries to hit my hand as though to remove or lower it; I let him do it and he grasps the box.

What shall we say about Laurent's behaviour at 7½ months, when he strikes his father's hand out of the way so that he can reach the matchbox that is the object of his interest? Certainly, we are inclined to call it an action. Although Laurent, who has not yet uttered his first words, would not be able to offer us reasons, we are nevertheless very likely to attribute intentionality to his movements. Is it an aggressive action? Again, Laurent cannot tell us what he intended, but I think that most of us would see his action as aimed at getting the matchbox, rather than hurting his father's hand. Thus, I think that most of us would reject the idea that Laurent's action was aggressive. Even if his movements had caused his father real pain, I think we would simply say that the injury was accidental. We do not attribute the capacity for aggression to an infant of this age.

Because almost everyone would be likely to agree that Marian and David's actions were aggressive, whereas Laurent's were not, these examples raise important questions: When and how does the capacity for aggressive action first emerge? How, and to what extent, do the frequency and character of aggression change during the course of development? Why? In the following section, the research literature is examined in an effort to address these questions.

Developmental Trends

One of the earliest studies of the origins of aggression was that of Goodenough, who drew her evidence from diaries kept by mothers of children ranging from 1 to 7 years of age. She found that, in terms of sheer frequencies, angry outbursts were most common among 1- to 2-year-olds. At 18 months, the children in her study averaged about one such outburst for every 6 hours they were awake. Three- and 4-year-olds, in contrast, showed only about half as many.

This finding does not, however, mean that these 1- and 2-year-olds were highly aggressive. The great majority of their outbursts of anger were not focused on any particular person or object. Most of these outbursts were, rather, what Maccoby has called "undirected tantrums," characterized by screaming, crying, and violent motor behaviour, but not, apparently, by any identifiable aggressive intent. On the other hand, focused outbursts of anger, such as those occurring in retaliation for a perceived injury, more than quadrupled from the 1- and 2-year-old period to the 3- and 4-year-old group. Thus, the appropriate conclusion to be drawn from Goodenough's findings would seem to be that although the incidence of violent and/or aversive behaviour reported by mothers declined after the age of 2, the incidence of reported aggression increased, at least up to 4 years of age.

Similar findings emerged from a study by Dawe. Drawing on observations of naturally occurring quarrels in a nursery school environment, Dawe reported that although preschoolers (54-65 months of age) were likely to respond to conflict with physical aggression such as pushing or hitting, toddlers (18-29 months) were more likely to exhibit what she called "undirected energy," including "crying, screaming, jumping up and down or stamping, without any directed resistance". It is worth noting that this latter category, although it includes much that is forceful or violent in nature, and much that would be aversive to almost any observer, nevertheless does not qualify as aggression in our terms. The results of Dawe's study are thus consistent with those of Goodenough in suggesting an increase in aggressive action, as such, over the preschool years.

There is a paradox of sorts in citing Dawe's findings to support the idea that aggression increases in frequency during the preschool years, because Dawe also reported that the frequency of conflicts between children decreases during this period. In her study, toddlers (18-29 months) were much more likely to start a quarrel, and in fact were involved in conflicts almost twice as often as older children (54-65 months). How can toddlers start more conflicts and quarrel more often, yet be less aggressive than preschool children? How can we account for this apparent discrepancy?

The answer lies in an examination of the nature of children's conflicts. The largest number of conflicts, at all of the ages Dawe studied, were those over objects. Among toddlers, object-centred quarrels accounted for almost three quarters of all observed conflict. The proportion of disputes that were centered on objects declined steadily with age, accounting for less than 40% of conflicts by the age of 5 years. In contrast, the proportion of conflict instigated by physical violence or disagreements over social rules showed marked increases over this same age period. In short, although preschoolers' conflicts were more likely to begin over physical violence or verbal disagreements, toddlers' disputes were more likely to start over possession of objects.

There is, in fact, good agreement among a variety of investigators that toddlers are particularly likely to experience conflict with their peers over objects. In the recent Hay and Ross study, for example, conflicts between pairs of 21 month-old children were recorded, and 84% of them proved to be struggles over toys.

If we were to imagine a prototypic object struggle between a pair of young toddlers, it might go something like this: One child (call her Marcy) is playing with a toy, a ball. Another child (call her Susan) notices the movements of the ball in Marcy's hands, becomes interested, and moves nearer. Susan reaches for the ball and takes it into her hands. In an effort to retrieve the ball again, Marcy runs into Susan, who pushes her away. Marcy loses her balance, falls, and begins to cry.

Now, the crucial question to ask about this episode is whether it is more like the encounter between David and Marian discussed earlier, or more like the one between Laurent and his father. In other words, is Susan's intention in this episode to be understood as "hurting Marcy" (and thus as aggressive like Marian) or as "getting the ball" (and hence as nonaggressive like Laurent)? It is often difficult to make this kind of judgment. When we watch episodes like this among young toddlers, however, I think we are most often inclined to see them as being more like Laurent's behaviour than like Marian's.

We are inclined to say that although Susan acted in such a way that the end result was painful to Marcy, this result was unexpected or accidental from Susan's point of view. Her intention was simply to get the ball, and she had little idea that the realization of her intention might prove painful to Marcy. Had Susan been an adult, we might be inclined to think that she should have foreseen at least some of these consequences, and so to hold her responsible. Because she is so young, however, we do not expect her to know these things, and we call her innocent. In fact, Levine has suggested that possessiveness and object struggles among toddlers stem more from the participants' emerging attempts at self-definition than from selfishness or aggressive intentions.

In these terms, then, what initially seemed to be a discrepancy in Dawe's findings that the incidence of aggression increased even as the frequency of conflict decreased during the preschool years appears instead to be exactly what we should expect. Very young children start more quarrels because they have no idea that their desire to manipulate interesting objects may have aversive consequences for their peers. Acting in complete, or near-complete, innocence, they are simply pursuing their own aims as best they can. Unaware of the potential ramifications of their actions for others, young toddlers often precipitate conflict, but may still remain incapable of aggression.

These early conflicts between peers must, however, have important implications for the emergence of aggression among children. If we imagine Susan's encounter with Marcy to be literally the first of its kind that she has experienced, then we must also imagine that Susan is in some way surprised at its outcome. With repeated experiences of this kind, however, Susan will learn that her peers do not like to have toys taken away from them, that they are likely to attempt retrieval of toys she has snatched, that struggle and injury may ensue, and so on. She will learn what neither she nor Laurent can initially be credited with knowing: that if, for whatever reason, she hits another person, it may hurt them. In short, she will learn that she is able to hurt others and in what ways, and this knowledge in turn will make it possible for her to act aggressively if and when she chooses to do so in the future. In other words, the knowledge she acquires in this way will create for her the possibility of aggressive action.

In this view, the emergence of a capacity for aggressive action action that is intended to hurt another person—is a momentous event, one that is dependent on cognitive achievements of a sophisticated nature. Drawing on Maccoby's discussion, we might say that the emergence of a capacity for true aggression requires, at a minimum, the understanding that there is a distinction between self and others; that others can experience distress; that one's own actions can cause distress in particular people; and that the execution of specific actions is likely to cause distress in a specific case. As Maccoby has stressed, the word "understanding" should be taken in a broad sense here; a child need not be able to recite a list of this sort in order to act in accordance with aggressive intentions. Still, it is clear that a capacity for aggressive action requires substantial cognitive development and learning; hence, this capacity might be expected to increase during the early childhood years. This view is very much in accord with the findings of what is perhaps the best known study of the development of aggression in childhood, that of Hartup.

Hartup's study involved observations of preschool (4- to 6-year-old) and elementary school (6- to 7-year-old) children's activities in their normal school environments. Aggressive events were defined as "intentional physical and verbal responses that are directed toward an object or another person and that have the capacity to damage or injure", and observers recorded all cases of such activities witnessed during a 10-week period. These were, in turn, divided into categories that Hartup called *instrumental aggression*, violent actions that are "aimed at the retrieval of an object, territory, or privilege"; and *hostile aggression*, violent actions that are aimed directly at harming or injuring another person. He also distinguished between verbal aggression (e.g., derogation, threats) and physical aggression (e.g., pushing, shoving).

Hartup's findings were these: Consistent with the results reported by Dawe, older children were more likely to respond to insults verbally, whereas younger children were more likely to respond with physical aggression. In other words, the extent to which apparently aggressive intentions were carried out verbally increased with age. In addition, elementary school children were less aggressive per unit time than were preschool children, and this decline was attributable to a decrease in "instrumental aggression." A significantly higher proportion of older children's aggression was hostile in nature. These findings are often cited as evidence for the proposition that instrumental aggression declines with age during this period.

To put these findings in the context that has been used here, some efforts at translation are required. We can start by recalling the distinction made earlier between aggression as such and the more general category of violent and/or aversive behaviour. Violent actions that are carried out with the intention of hurting another person are those we have termed aggressive. Those carried out for some other reason (e.g., to retrieve an object, as in the example of Laurent, or in that of Susan and Marcy) we called violent and/or aversive, but not aggressive. In our terms, then, the concept of "instrumental aggression" aggression that is *not* aimed at hurting another person is a misnomer, a contradiction in terms.

In our terms, what Hartup has called "instrumental aggression" is simply violent or aversive action undertaken to achieve some nonaggressive goal, such as the retrieval of an object. As adults, we may be tempted to label this an aggressive activity because if we undertook it, we would do so in anticipation of its hurtful consequences for another person. To the extent that we believe young children are without such anticipation, however, we cannot be justified in labeling their actions as aggressive; to do so would be no more than the projection of our own preoccupations onto them.

In summary, Hartup's findings seem to show both a greater frequency of true aggression and a greater reluctance to use violent means to non-hostile ends among elementary school as compared to preschool children. As such, his observations are consistent with, and also extend those of Goodenough and Dawe. Thus, the most important conclusion emerging from these findings seems to be that, as they get older, children increasingly confine their use of physical violence to their pursuit of aggressive aims.

An important qualification to this conclusion, however, is that it rests on our interpretations of children's intentions. The meanings of actions are given by our interpretations of them, and our interpretations are always subject to disagreement, discussion, and debate. Thus, although we may be inclined to interpret some of children's actions as aggressive and others as nonaggressive, we should do so only in recognition that other interpretations are also possible. When we are concerned with the actions of adults, our respect for the potential range and complexity of underlying intentions makes this recognition relatively easy to achieve. Even when they seem most transparent, however, the actions of children are worthy of our respect in this regard as well. Overall, then, confidence in our conclusions should be tempered by acknowledgment of the primacy of ambiguity in the interpretation of human actions.

With this qualification in mind, we can summarize the tentative conclusions that we have reached. In the behaviour of infants and very young children, it appears that violence and aggression are often distinguishable; physically violent behaviour frequently occurs without aggressive intent. Increasingly with age, however, physical violence and aggression do appear to become almost interchangeable terms in practice, inasmuch as older children increasingly seem to use violent means only when their goals are aggressive. Thus, during the early childhood period, there appears to be both an increasing capacity to conceive and carry out aggressive intentions as well as a growing association of physical violence with aggressive intent in children's activities. What might account for these trends?

Underlying Factors

It has been said that even to conceive an aggressive intention is a sophisticated cognitive achievement. Certainly, then, it must represent an even more sophisticated achievement to limit the use of violence and aversive techniques to those cases in which our intentions are actually to harm. What underlies these achievements? We can begin our discussion of these questions by considering an episode related by Maccoby: "During a long ride in the car, a four-year-old boy lay down on the car seat with his head in his mother's lap. He gazed deeply into his mother's eyes. The mother felt pleased at this loving intimacy. Then the boy said, "Mom, your eyes are just like road-maps!".

This remark, if made by an adult, might well be considered an insult; it might be interpreted as a deliberate attempt to hurt the woman's feelings or injure her pride. In other words, it might be considered aggressive. As Maccoby explains, however, "The mother was not pleased, of course, to have attention called to her bloodshot eyes. But she understood that the child did not intend to hurt her feelings." In other words, the remark could not be considered aggressive, because the little boy did not understand how his remark would make his mother feel.

As this episode suggests, efforts to comprehend the development of aggression must take into account the growth of social understanding. As I have argued, it is the growth of social understanding that makes aggression possible; certainly, the growth of social understanding can also help to explain the changes in its forms with advancing age. Let us look, then, at some of the evidence on how social understanding in particular, the appreciation of social perspectives other than one's own seems to affect the development of aggression.

It is an interesting but regrettable fact that research on the social understanding of aggression and violence tends to begin with children of elementary school age. Among older children, victims' interpretations of perpetrators' intentions clearly influence their responses to violence. For example, highly aggressive children are more likely than their less aggressive peers to interpret the behaviour of others as stemming from hostile intentions. Both aggressive and nonaggressive children are more likely to retaliate in kind if they believe themselves to be the victims of intentional, as opposed to accidental, violence.

It would be useful, then, to know how very young children interpret their playmates' attempts to take toys from them. Do they regard these actions as instrumental, or as hostile? Does it matter? When one toddler inadvertently pushes or injures another in the midst of a dispute, is this regarded by the victim as accidental or intentional? And how does this affect the victim's response? There is little information available with which to answer such questions.

There is some suggestion in the literature that preschool children may interpret any of another person's movements as intentional. Smith showed 4-, 5-, and 6-year-old children videotaped sequences of adult behaviour and asked them to judge its degree of intentionality (i.e., the extent to which the actor was trying, or wanted, to do the particular behaviour displayed on the videotape). He found that 4-year-olds tended to regard almost all movements, even involuntary ones such as sneezing, as intentional activity. Even very undesirable effects (e.g., garbage landing on the floor instead of in the garbage can), labelled by adults as unintended, were perceived as intended by 4-year-olds. Older children, particularly 6-year-olds, recognized that even though an action might be voluntary, all of its effects might not be intended.

Smith's findings may have important implications for understanding the development of aggression because they suggest that young children may regard any outcome they encounter at the hands of their peers, no matter how negative or aversive, as intended. To the extent that young children are biased to view any effects of a person's actions as intended, they must also often overestimate the extent to which their peers' intentions are hostile. Hence, they may see their peers as more hostile than they "really are" (i.e., more hostile than adult observers would believe them to be). Such an attributional bias might increase young children's likelihood of responding to accidental violence with real aggression, and so lead to the needless escalation of many conflicts. If correct, this line of reasoning would seem partly to account for the relatively high frequencies of conflicts that begin in the context of object struggles among younger children. In the absence of relevant data, however, these suggestions remain entirely speculative.

Research on children's ability to differentiate intentional from unintentional violence in the behaviour of their peers does not begin until school age. Shantz and Voydanoff told boys stories about another boy who committed some violent acts, thereby harming another child. In some stories, the violence was intentional (i.e., aggressive); in others, it was unintentional (i.e., accidental). The boys were asked to choose among different levels of physical punishment for the child who had been violent. The major finding was that while 9- and 12-year olds chose less severe punishment for the accidental acts of violence, 7-year-olds did not differentiate between accidental and intentional (i.e., truly aggressive) violence.

In contrast, Dodge reports that 7-year-old boys did make such a distinction. In Dodge's study, boys worked on a puzzle, which was subsequently spoiled, either accidentally or on purpose, by another boy. They subsequently had an opportunity either to help or to hurt the child who had spoiled their work. Seven-year-olds showed a greater tendency to hurt, physically as well as verbally, the child who had spoiled their work on purpose. The discrepancy between Dodge's findings and those of Shantz and Voydanoff might be attributed to any of a number of procedural differences between the two studies, or it might reflect a genuine instability in children's responses at this age; further research is necessary to resolve this point.

In a related study, Ferguson and Rule have shown that by the age of eight, boys held an actor more responsible (i.e., said that the actor was more to blame) for the negative consequences of his violent behaviour when they were intended than when they were not. In addition, the oldest boys (14-year-olds) not only put more blame on the actor for the intended than for the unintended negative effects of his actions, but they also differentiated between accidental but-foreseeable versus accidental-and-not-foreseeable negative effects, attributing more blame for the former than the latter. Eight-year-olds did not make this distinction. Thus, older children apparently expect their peers to make reasonable efforts to foresee the probable consequences of their actions, and to take them into account. To the extent that the actor did not behave in these ways, and to the extent that the effects of his actions on others were negative, he was considered blameworthy by older, but not younger, children.

In a further study by Rule, Nesdale, and McAra, children were asked to attribute blame for intentionally violent and/ or aversive actions that were committed with hostile (angry), personal-instrumental (selfish), or social-instrumental (prosocial) intentions. In one study, 5-year-old girls labelled those actions committed with hostile intentions as more reprehensible than those performed with social-instrumental intentions. In another, 6-year-old boys called actions committted for hostile or selfish motives more reprehensible than those undertaken for prosocial purposes. It is interesting to note that personal-instrumental intentions were treated by 6-year-olds in essentially the same way as hostile ones. This finding seems consistent with the suggestion from Smith's study that young children may be likely to over-attribute intentionality to actions and their effects.

In general, the available research seems to reveal children's increasing sensitivity with age to the varying intentions that underlie the particular behaviours they observe. Although the available evidence is still fragmentary in nature, it appears that over the preschool and early elementary school years, children may become less likely to over-attribute hostile intent in the behaviour of others, and more likely to recognize alternative interpretations. Thus, the decrease during this period in the frequency of peer conflicts that begin in the context of object struggles may be explained, at least in part, by developments in the social cognitive domain.

Whereas children seem to become less likely with age to attribute hostile intentions to their peers when these attributions are not justified, they may also become more likely to notice and respond to cues of actual hostility from their peers. For instance, by the age of about 6 years, children are able to identify those facial expressions that signify their peers' unwillingness to give up possession of contested objects, and to name the emotional states portrayed by those expressions. Even 5-year-olds adjusted their behaviour in disputes appropriately when their peers exhibited facial expressions of antagonism; children at this age were less likely to persist in their attempts to take possession of a desired object when a peer produced antagonistic expressions than when a peer produced more neutral facial cues while defending his or her possession of a disputed object.

It would be interesting to compare the responses of younger children in situations similar to those Camras studied. Judging from the frequency of toddlers' object-related disputes with their peers, we might expect them to be somewhat less adept at reading a peer's nonverbal signs of imminent retaliation. Very young children might also be less likely than preschoolers and elementary school children to adjust their own actions before the conflict has escalated.

Until relevant data on younger children become available, however, this possibility cannot be evaluated.

By the age of 5 or 6 years children seem to understand at least some aspects of their peers' expressive behaviour signalling the likelihood of resistance or compliance with their own assertive maneuvers. Children at this age also seem to be highly responsive to the degree of success or failure they experience in specific peer encounters. For example, Patterson, Littman and Bricker observed peer conflicts in nursery schools and reported that children were less likely to initiate conflicts with peers who had retaliated successfully against them in previous encounters. To the extent that physically violent methods were unsuccessful in achieving their aims, these children increasingly turned either to other victims or to alternative forms of behaviour.

Taken together, the results of the Camras and Patterson studies suggest that during the late preschool and early elementary school periods, children may become increasingly sensitive to their peers' often unfavourable responses to physically violent behaviour. To the extent that children of this age have learned that victims of their violent actions may retaliate, and to the extent that they have also learned to read the nonverbal signs of imminent retaliation, they might well be expected to begin to search in earnest for nonviolent methods of achieving their non-hostile (e.g., instrumental) aims. Thus, the trend during this age period for children increasingly to confine their use of violent methods to their achievement of hostile aims may be partially explained by data such as these.

Summary

The frequency of verbal aggression increases markedly during this age period, while the frequency of physical aggression appears to drop. Thus, the major developmental achievement of early childhood in this regard appears to be an increasing ability to confine the use of physical violence to the pursuit of hostile aims and to develop alternative means of achieving other, non-hostile aims. Both children's increasing levels of social understanding in general and their actual experience with peers in particular seem to underlie these developmental trends.

Emergence and Development of Altruistic Action

Just as we earlier recognized a distinction between antisocial behaviour and aggressive action, so we need also to distinguish between prosocial behaviour and altruistic action. Prosocial behaviour that has the effect of benefitting or sustaining others is a large and ramified category. Altruistic action prosocial behaviour that is undertaken *with the intention of* providing such benefits to others is a subset of this category.

Prosocial behaviour includes not only such paradigm cases as contributing to charities and rescuing victims of disasters, but also a host of other everyday, conventional activities that result in benefits to others. When we operate automobiles in accordance with local traffic ordinances we contribute to the safety and welfare of others who use the same highways. When we conform to prevailing customs of dress, manners, and conduct, we benefit those around us by providing them with a relatively stable, predictable environment in which to pursue their own daily activities. When we comply with the conventions of conversation and discourse indeed, of languages themselves we benefit others by facilitating communication, and so rendering the pursuit of joint activities easier. It is difficult to overestimate the depth and range of the influence of convention in our lives, and it is more difficult still to overestimate the benefits that accrue to us as a result. Thus, a very large proportion of our normal, everyday activities can be considered prosocial behaviour.

Although many of our everyday activities have beneficial effects on others, a much smaller proportion of them are undertaken with the intention of having these effects. When we fit our activities to the requirements of local traffic laws, customs of dress, or conventions of conversation, we most often do so almost without thinking. When we do think about such matters, most of us probably think first about our own self-interest. For instance, when we are deciding whether or not to drive in excess of posted speed limits, most of us probably evaluate first the probability of getting a speeding ticket, not the probability of injuring other drivers. Thus, while many of our activities have prosocial effects, only a small proportion of them can be classified as altruistic actions.

The ability to act in an altruistic manner involves not only the ability to distinguish between self and other, but also the knowledge that people might need help, that some kinds of events or conditions are likely to help them, and that certain kinds of actions are likely to bring about the relevant events or conditions. It also involves the ability and desire to carry out such actions in specific cases. An altruistic act, then, is a complex cognitive achievement. When and how does the capacity for altruistic action emerge in the normal course of development? And how does it change during the course of childhood? In this section, the research evidence is examined for answers to these questions.

Developmental Trends

We begin by considering the following report from a longitudinal study conducted by Radke-Yarrow and Zahn-Waxler: a child at 12 months, when confronted with a peer's cries, responds with a primitive distress cry of her own and turns to her mother to be nestled and stroked. A few weeks later, when her mother has scalded her hand, the child cries, nestles into her mother but also hugs her mother now giving some comfort as well as getting comfort. At 17 months, in the presence of a crying baby, her expression is concerned and tearful, but she strokes the baby's head, hugs and pats him, offers toys, and finally tries to bring her mother to the rescue.

This account of one child's development over a period of only a few months is interesting in a number of different ways. Radke-Yarrow and her colleagues do not provide us with this little girl's name, but let us call her Jessica. At 12 months, Jessica cries in response to the cries of a peer. She does not seem to differentiate herself from the other, and perhaps is therefore unable to offer comfort to the other child. Within a few weeks, however, she manages to combine her own desire for comfort upon noticing her mother's distress, with the possibility of offering her mother a hug as well. By the age of 17 months, Jessica is able to differentiate her own concern from that of the baby, and manages both to conceive and to carry out at least four different strategies to calm the baby's distress.

Of course, no brief excerpt can offer us all of the information that we might like, and the interpretation of this one is certainly open to question. Even granting that Jessica's behaviour at 17 months appears intentional, we may still remain uncertain about her motives. Was her main aim to reduce the baby's distress? Or was her principal concern rather to eliminate unpleasant auditory stimulation from her own environment? Answers to these questions are by no means clear. On the basis of the information contained in this excerpt, however, many of us would probably be inclined to label 17-month-old Jessica's actions toward the baby as altruistic.

How is it possible that a child as young as 17 months could manage the complex cognitive tasks, upon the mastery of which we have said that altruistic action depends? The achievement is enormous, and nothing should detract from our amazement that such a young child should prove able to make it. This being said, however, it is also worth noting several factors which combine to make Jessica's situation seem particularly favourable. First, her mother (who made the observation) was present; Jessica's own level of psychological comfort or security was therefore probably relatively high when the baby began to cry. Second, it seems likely, given what we know of toddlers' lives, that the crying baby was a familiar person, perhaps even a sibling. Third, the other's distress was very clearly signaled by the baby's apparently loud and persistent crying. Finally, the kinds of actions needed in order to implement an altruistic intention (e.g., making physical contact, offering toys) were familiar and well-practiced elements of Jessica's pre-existing behavioural repertoire.

Although all four of these factors are probably relevant to the 17-month-old's ability to undertake altruistic action, I focus here on research which bears on the last two only. The available evidence clearly suggests developmental trends in both children's ability to identify cues of distress in other people, and in the size and complexity of the behavioural repertoires available to them for responding to any perceived needs for altruistic action. I first describe some of the research findings on infants and very young children, and then turn to the evidence relevant to preschool and elementary school children.

Negative responding to certain very clear signs of another's distress seems to be present essentially from birth. Simner, as well as Sagi and Hoffman have reported that the vocal properties of another baby's cries seem to promote crying in newborn infants. In the Simner study, for example, infants were more likely to cry when they heard a tape recording of another newborn's cry than when they heard white noise, or no noise, or indeed, a computer simulation of a newborn's cry. We are, of course, not likely on this basis to credit the newborn with a capacity for altruistic action. Reports such as these do, however, provide evidence of a particular sensitivity to signs of distress in others very early in life.

Similar accounts of older infants' and toddlers' distress in response to crying in peers also exist. Hay, Nash, and Pederson failed to find moment-to moment correspondence between the crying patterns of 6-month-old playmates, but did report evidence that one infant's crying had cumulative effects on a peer of the same age. Especially when there were no potentially distracting toys available in the infants' environment, the conditional probability of one infant's crying, given that the other had been crying, increased dramatically over intervals of time as short as 30 seconds. Crying in response to the distress of a peer has also been reported among 1- and 2-year-olds.

There is also evidence that infants can discriminate among a variety of different facial expressions (see Bornstein, in this volume). For example, Buhler and Hetzer found that infants are able to discriminate angry and smiling faces by the age of about six or seven months. These reports have been confirmed by La Barbera, Izard, Vietze and Parisi, as well as by Wilcox and Clayton. Cohn and Tronick have recently reported that 3-month-olds respond differently when their mothers show depressed, as opposed to normal affect. Studies of early language use offer convergent evidence on this point; soon after children learn to speak, their utterances seem to reflect comprehension of the meanings of various facial expressions such as those associated with sadness.

By the age of two, then, most children must be capable of discriminating and responding to a variety of relatively clear expressions of distress in the people around them. A marked tendency to react with distress to the cries of others appears much earlier. To the extent that this kind of responsiveness can be taken as evidence for the existence of an empathic predisposition, the available evidence suggests that such a predisposition is either present very early in life, or develops quite rapidly during the first several months.

A limited repertoire of cooperative and other prosocial behaviours also seems to be well-established by the end of infancy. For example, Hay studied early forms of cooperation and sharing among 12-, 18-, and 24-month-olds as they played in the presence of their parents. At 12 months, almost every child was observed to show objects to others, and half also gave objects to parents during play. At 18 months, all the children both showed and gave toys. Rheingold, Hay, and West studied 15- to 18-month-olds in similar situations ; they reported that all babies demonstrated forms of prosocial behaviour, such as the giving and showing of objects, and that most shared not only with their parents, but also with unfamiliar adults. Similar observations of early sharing and cooperative behaviour have also been made by others.

A particularly interesting study in this vein was reported by Rheingold. Children at 18, 24, and 30 months were observed while their parents or other adults carried out a number of common household chores (e.g., folding laundry, sweeping, setting a table). In spite of the fact that the adults did not ask for assistance, all of the children did in fact offer help. Sixty-five per cent of the 18 month-olds, 95% of the 24-month-olds, and all of the 30-month-olds helped on more than half of the tasks their parents performed. Thus, not only did the majority of children participate in their parents' work, most offered assistance on the majority of tasks. Almost all of the children also participated in the work performed by unfamiliar adults. While the children sometimes imitated their parents' behaviour, they also went beyond simple imitation in their efforts to complete tasks (e.g., by placing bits of paper onto a dustpan by hand when they were not able to do this using a broom).

One intriguing aspect of Rheingold's findings was that the children's efforts were sometimes accompanied by their utterance of intention statements (e.g., "fold clothes"; "I'm going to pick up these books") and/or by their signalling verbally when a task had been completed (e.g., "all clean"; "I'm all through with my little broom"). The frequency of these utterances increased with the age of the child, but even the 18-month-olds offered some remarks of this sort. As Rheingold notes, verbalizations like these do not prove that the children intended to be helpful. They are interesting, however, because they seem to provide evidence of the children's awareness of their contributions to the completion of joint tasks, and because they therefore raise at least the possibility that these children's activities may not have been merely prosocial, but altruistic as well.

In a longitudinal study, Radke-Yarrow and Zahn-Waxler (in press) trained mothers to record instances of their children's prosocial behaviour over a period of 9 months. On the basis of the mothers' observations, Radke-Yarrow and Zahn Waxler reported that, even by 10 to 12 months, children responded with some regularity to evidence of distress in others. The most frequent response at this age was "a frown, a sad face, cries, and/or visual checking with the caregiver". By 18 to 24 months, children's responses often included physical contact and positive initiations to the distressed person. By the age of two, children began to bring objects to the individual in distress, verbalize sympathy, make suggestions, and bring somebody else to help. They also began to try alternative strategies if an initial attempt at providing comfort failed. Not all of the children's responses were positive or prosocial in nature; in a small minority of instances, children attempted to avoid, escape, or even attack a person in distress. Overall, although the results do not permit unambiguous interpretation in terms of altruism, they are at least consistent with the idea that there is a substantial expansion during the second year in children's repertoires for prosocial behaviour.

By the age of three, then, most children seem able to discriminate and comprehend some of the major expressions of negative emotion in others and to respond to them in a variety of appropriate ways. They also seem, at least sometimes, to be motivated to share, to reduce the distress, and to participate in the activities of the people around them. Further, they are often capable of doing these things. We turn now to the further developments that take place as children grow older.

One such area of development involves children's ability to recognize relatively subtle cues of another person's distress. In a study by Pearl, 4- and 8-year-olds were exposed to videotaped scenes in which a child had difficulty in performing a task. When cues to the actor's distress were highly salient and explicit, younger children were as likely to recognize distress as older children. When the cues were more subtle, however, young children were less likely to infer sadness or frustration, whereas older children continued to do so. In their longitudinal study of children from 2 to 7 years of age, Radke-Yarrow and Zahn Waxler (in press) also found that older children seemed responsive to a wider range of cues to distress. When one considers the variety of subtle and often indirect ways in which both children and adults may signal distress, it seems likely that we still have much to learn about the development of the ability to recognize these signals.

It has often been suggested that, throughout the preschool and elementary school years, the frequency of prosocial behaviour increases with age. As Radke-Yarrow and her colleagues have suggested, however, this proposition is in need of close scrutiny. Although, as we have already seen, there is evidence for increases in the frequency of prosocial behaviour during early childhood, no such simple trend seems to characterize changes during the middle or later years of childhood. After reviewing the results of over 75 different studies, Radke-Yarrow and her colleagues concluded that "the data from existing research do not support a simple unidirectional trend". As these authors have pointed out, when one considers the enormous array of diverse activities that might be included under the rubric of prosocial behaviour, particularly for older children, this conclusion should perhaps not seem surprising.

Although the actual frequency of prosocial behaviour probably does not increase during middle and later childhood, there is some evidence that the size and adequacy of children's repertoires of skills for prosocial action does expand. A fascinating glimpse of the possibilities here is provided in a study by Burleson. In this study, first- through twelfth-graders were asked to respond to hypothetical situations in which a same-sex peer was experiencing distress; each child was asked to describe all of the ways in which he or she might be able to offer comfort in each of four different situations. The main findings were that the size and diversity of children's repertoires of comforting strategies grew with age, and that the rated quality of the strategies they suggested improved with age also. For instance, first graders were more likely to suggest strategies that involved denial of the feelings of the distressed other, whereas older children more often sought to acknowledge and to legitimize the peer's perspective. Thus, Burleson's results suggest that, at least in the domain of verbal comforting skills, children's repertoires for altruistic action do increase with age.

In summary, the evidence reviewed suggests that the predisposition to react negatively to clear signs of others' distress exists very early in life, that the ability to conceive and carry out altruistic actions may emerge at some time during the second year, and that the frequency and variety of prosocial behaviour increases after that time up until the age of about 3 or 4 years. Although prosocial behaviour does not seem to increase in frequency after the age of about 4 years, there is some evidence suggesting that the ability to recognize cues of distress improves and that the repertoire of behavioural strategies for accomplishing altruistic aims expands during the course of middle and later childhood. What factors might explain these trends?

Underlying Factors

A number of hypotheses about possible factors underlying the observed trends have been advanced. These include explanations based on concepts as diverse as guilt, intelligence, perspective-taking skill, and empathy.

Although there has been little systematic research on the first two topics, a considerable body of data has accumulated with respect to the latter two concepts. A substantial amount of research has also been directed to the relationship between children's reasoning about and actual performance of prosocial behaviour.

Although no investigator has suggested that any unidimensional explanation can account for the full range of developmental phenomena in this area, empirical studies often tend to focus on the relationships between children's prosocial behaviour and one or two measures of an explanatory concept of interest. The specific measures of both prosocial behaviour itself and the constructs entertained as possible mediators of this behaviour vary widely among studies. It is perhaps for this reason that research findings are often disparate and difficult to evaluate.

As an example, consider the research on relationships between perspective taking skill and prosocial behaviour. The principal prediction here is that improvements in the ability to appreciate others' perspectives should be associated with increased tendencies to act in a prosocial manner. Measures of perspective taking have included social, affective, cognitive, and perceptual tasks; measures of prosocial behaviour have typically assessed either sharing or helping, but these have, of course, been defined differently in different studies. Some investigators have found the expected positive relationships; others have not. Some findings have been mixed. The situation with regard to research on empathy and children's prosocial behaviour is very similar. On the basis of the existing evidence, definitive conclusions on these issues do not seem warranted.

Although research on the role of perspective taking and empathy has not yet proven conclusive, studies of children's conceptions of and reasoning about prosocial behaviour have been illuminating. In particular, studies have examined children's reasoning about their own prosocial behaviour, as well as their conceptions about the behaviour of their peers. We briefly consider some of the results of this research.

A number of investigators have asked children to explain the reasons for their own prosocial behaviour. The general finding has been that when children are questioned about their motives for particular prosocial behaviours, such as instances of sharing or helping, they are most likely to explain them by referring to what might be called sociocentric intentions. Although young children also give reasons based on pragmatic considerations (e.g., their own qualifications as helpers), even among preschoolers explanations that focus on the needs of other people are among the most common responses. Reasoning that focuses on altruistic motives for prosocial behaviour increases in frequency with age.

Notably absent from the reasoning of even the youngest children tested in this research (viz., 4-year-olds) are explanations of their own prosocial behaviour by reference to the demands of authority figures or to the desire to avoid punishment. This latter finding is particularly interesting in light of the prevalence of authority and punishment-oriented reasoning in young children's responses to questions about moral transgressions. When young children are asked their reasons for avoiding transgressions, they often focus on manifestly selfish motives (e.g., the desire to avoid punishment); when they are asked their reasons for performing prosocial behaviour such as sharing, on the other hand, they often focus on apparently altruistic intentions (e.g., the desire to satisfy another's needs). In short, the interpretations of their own prosocial behaviour offered even by preschool children are often made in terms of what seem to be altruistic motives.

Eisenberg-Berg and her colleagues have also investigated the development of reasoning about prosocial behaviour in the context of hypothetical dilemmas. For example, Eisenberg-Berg and Hand found that preschoolers used principally hedonistic (i.e., selfish) and needs-oriented (i.e., altruistic) reasoning when explaining their choices in hypothetical prosocial moral conflicts. When the same children were re-tested 18 months later, they demonstrated more needs-oriented and less hedonistic reasoning. Older children show continuing decreases in immature forms of reasoning, such as hedonistic reasoning, and increases in more mature (e.g., abstract and/or internalized) forms.

The relationships between prosocial moral reasoning on hypothetical dilemmas and prosocial behaviour among young children have also been studied. Eisenberg-Berg and Hand found that 4-year-olds' frequency of sharing with other children in their nursery school was positively related to the incidence of needs-oriented reasoning, and negatively related to the incidence of hedonistic reasoning that they demonstrated in response to prosocial moral dilemmas. Examining this general relationship in more detail, the authors discovered that it was attributable to the correlations between children's reasoning and their spontaneous sharing in the nursery school environment; children's sharing in response to requests from their peers was unrelated to their reasoning on the prosocial dilemmas. As Eisenberg-Berg and Hand have noted, these findings "are consistent with the conclusion that sharing in response to a request may be motivated by less altruistic considerations than is spontaneous sharing." Thus, as these authors suggested, the results of this research serve to emphasize that it is "important to consider the motivations underlying behaviours that superficially appear to involve altruism."

Finally, there has also been some research on the development of children's attributions of kindness in the behaviour of others. The most interesting finding here has been that, when judging the kindness of another person's actions, young children (e.g., kindergartners) do not seem to discriminate between intentional and unintentional behaviour. By second grade, however, this distinction is crucial to children's attributions of kindness. When these results are considered along with Smith's finding that young children regard a much wider array of behaviours as intentional than do older children or adults, they again serve to underscore the way in which children's understanding of intentionality can affect their interpretations of prosocial behaviour.

The overall yield of research on factors underlying developmental trends in children's prosocial behaviour, and in children's interpretation of the prosocial behaviour of others, has been uneven. Although there has been a great deal of research in some areas, and much less in others, the strength of the conclusions that seem to be warranted in any particular area bears little relation to the amount of research. The clearest findings show that even young children frequently offer interpretations of their own prosocial behaviour in terms of motives that might be considered altruistic, that there are reliable developmental trends in reasoning about prosocial behaviour, and that these trends appear to be related to children's actual behaviour. It also seems to be true that, in comparison with older children and adults, young children may often over-attribute altruistic intentions in the prosocial behaviour of others.

Summary

The results of research on the emergence and development of altruistic action suggest a number of interrelated conclusions. First, the predisposition to react negatively to clear signs of another's distress appears to exist very early in infancy. It seems reasonable to assume that such a predisposition might give rise to altruistic aims quite early in life, and the available data, although still very scanty, are consistent with this view; the earliest manifestations of truly altruistic actions seem to emerge at some point during the second year. At this time, children's ability to separate their own from another's distress become sufficient to allow them to generate responses that might be expected to reduce the other's distress. As one might expect, however, the 2-year-old's repertoire for altruistic action remains quite limited.

The frequency and variety of prosocial behaviour seem to increase up until the age of about 3 or 4 years. After that time, significant developments take place both in the ability to recognise relatively subtle cues of distress in others, and in the size of children's behavioural repertoires for responding to such distress, but not, apparently, in the actual frequency with which children exhibit prosocial behaviour. Whether the frequency of altruistic action per se changes during this period cannot be determined on the basis of available evidence. The data do, however, suggest that there are significant changes in children's reasoning about prosocial episodes with age and that these are related to children's actual performance of prosocial behaviour.

Aggression, Altruism and Self-Regulation in Childhood

As has already been said, self-regulation entails the successful achievement of personally selected aims or goals. As such, efforts to achieve self-regulation presuppose the existence of at least one goal or intention to be realized through action, and they involve the selection, from an available repertoire, of those actions which are expected to result in achievement of that goal. Thus, both the emergence of the aims themselves and the creation of a repertoire of strategies for achieving these aims are important aspects of the development of self-regulation. Let us consider the development of aggression and altruism in these terms.

In developmental terms, the emergence of truly aggressive or altruistic aims is an important milestone. Although these intentions seem to appear very early in childhood, they nevertheless depend upon a number of cognitive achievements. Some of the cognitive prerequisites for the emergence of aggressive or altruistic action seem to be knowledge that the self can be differentiated from others, that other people can be hurt or helped, that particular kinds of conditions or events are particularly likely to hurt or help them, and that one's own behaviour can bring about these conditions or events. Thus, the first appearance of a truly aggressive or altruistic action presupposes the accomplishment of a number of sophisticated cognitive tasks; hence, it is an event of real developmental significance.

Having conceived an aggressive or an altruistic intention, a child immediately faces the problem of translating it into action. We have seen evidence of the growth of children's repertoires in this regard, both in the area of aggression (e.g., the increasing use of verbal skills in aggressive encounters among older children) and in the area of altruism (e.g., the development of the skills involved in comforting another person who is distressed). Growth in the size and accessibility of children's repertoires for aggressive and altruistic action is a major accomplishment of the childhood period.

Thus, both the emergence of aggressive and altruistic intentions and the creation of a repertoire of strategies for the implementation of these intentions in action are important aspects of the development of aggression and altruism during the childhood years. It is perhaps tempting to imagine that this is all that is involved in the development of aggressive and altruistic action in childhood. To do so, however, would be a mistake, for if we stop here, we may overlook one of the most interesting aspects of the topic the role of self-control. Before examining the contribution of self-control to changes in children's aggression and altruism with age, however, we need to pause briefly in order to consider, from a more general perspective, the relationship between self-control and self regulation.

It has been suggested that self-regulation involves the successful achievement of personally selected aims and goals, and that this means that the domain of self-regulation is essentially coterminous with the realm of effective, intentional action. What is perhaps most surprising about this realm is how many of our day-to-day activities it encompasses. In our normal, everyday lives as adults, for example, we go to bed at the hours of our own choosing at night, and arise at the times we deem appropriate in the morning; we dress ourselves, feed ourselves, and prepare ourselves for the anticipated events of the day. All of these activities, and countless others like them, however conventional or habitual they may have become, are done to realise personal intentions, and most often they are done successfully. What is first of all remarkable, then, is how effective our attempts at self-regulation normally seem to be, and how little effort they normally seem to require. Self-regulation is so ordinary that most of the time we scarcely even notice that it is taking place.

There are times, however, when something seems to go wrong. I find that I do not feel sleepy at the hour I have chosen as my bedtime, or that I am not ready to arise when my alarm rings in the morning. The clothes I had planned to wear turn out to be wrinkled or spotted; my favourite breakfast foods are missing from the refrigerator. At times such as these, the achievement of a goal is blocked, or the realization of one goal interferes with the achievement of another; effective self regulation is challenged. A problem emerges and the need for "self-control" becomes evident. It is a breakdown, or the threat of a breakdown, in the normal stream of self-regulated behaviour that makes what we call self-control seem necessary. Perhaps it is the very infrequency with which such problems arise that makes them seem so noticeable, so extraordinary, when they do.

Thus, one might think of self-control as the "figure" and self-regulation as the "ground" of voluntary activity. The need for self-control emerges only against a background of voluntary activity because it is only out of attempts to achieve personal goals that the possibility of failure in doing so could arise. It is only in the context of the belief that I normally, or at least sometimes, am in control of my actions that the possibility that I am not could seem problematic or threatening, or indeed have any meaning at all. It is only my normal ability to fit my actions easily to self-articulated intentions or rules that makes it seem remarkable when special efforts become necessary. Hence, the emergence of self control as an issue the very possibility of taking "extraordinary" measures to make my actions fit with pre-established intentions or rules depends on the "ordinary" ability to do so almost without thinking. One might say, then, that the problem of self-control rests on the assumption of self-regulation.

How, then, do problems of self-control arise in the context of children's aggressive and altruistic actions? One sort of threat to self-regulation occurs when a child wants to achieve a particular goal but does not know how to go about it. For instance, as has already been mentioned, a young child who wants to comfort a distressed adult may not have a repertoire of comforting skills that is adequate to the task. Threats to self-regulation can also stem from a situation in which the achievement of one aim is seen as interfering with the accomplishment of another. A child may want to achieve certain instrumental goals, such as the possession of desirable toys, may have available only physically violent methods with which to achieve these goals, and yet want also to maintain harmonious relations with peers. As other children tend to dislike peers who are considered aggressive, the child in this position may experience a conflict between attempts to achieve instrumental goals on the one hand, and efforts to accomplish social goals on the other.

As Maccoby has emphasized, physical violence "carries a high cost; it is painful to the aggressor, and it jeopardizes continued social contact." Thus, children who use violence to achieve their instrumental (e.g., non-hostile) aims do so at the risk of being disliked and so avoided by their victims. To the extent that these victims are part of the fabric of everyday life, the price of aggression for these children is ultimately the risk of severing social connections with the people around them. Since this is, of course, a very high price to pay, the recognition of a conflict between the use of violence to accomplish one's instrumental goals and the possibility of simultaneously achieving highly valued social goals might be expected to trigger a search for alternatives to violence. The recognition of a problem in self-regulation, in other words, might be expected to result in efforts at self-control. The developmental trends that characterize the period of early childhood, as we have seen, are consistent with the idea that most children arrive at something very much like this kind of recognition during this period.

What is important to notice here is that recognition of conflicts can pave the way for discovery of solutions. Until children become aware of a problem, they are not likely to make efforts to solve it. It is the recognition of a threat to self regulation that gives rise to efforts at self-control; it is the recognition of the difficulty in coordinating the simultaneous pursuit of more than one goal that gives rise to problem-solving attempts, and ultimately to the discovery of nonviolent methods of achieving instrumental aims. Thus, beginning to recognise conflicts of this kind is an important developmental step.

The recognition of conflicts between various goals requires that more than one goal be kept in mind at the same time, and this may be very difficult for the young child. As long as a child focuses attention on any one goal to the exclusion of others, conflicts arising in the coordination of goals will not be recognised. As we know from studies of cognitive development, there is enormous improvement during the early and middle childhood years in the ability to keep more than one concept in mind simultaneously. Thus, it is perhaps no coincidence that children's ability to limit their use of violence to the pursuit of aggressive aims expands dramatically during these years.

For a young child to notice and respond appropriately to conflicts among his or her various social and instrumental aims is a difficult cognitive achievement.

Because the task is so demanding, it is reasonable to assume that it might not be undertaken at all much less, successfully unless the conditions are relatively favourable. What circumstances might be expected to make this kind of task more or less accessible to a child?

As physical violence is a readily available aspect of the young child's behavioural repertoire and as overlearned responses are more likely than novel ones to be produced under stressful conditions, we might expect that in stressful circumstances, violent strategies would be the first to come to a child's mind. Certainly, the available evidence suggests this is the case throughout early childhood. Under conditions of lower stress, however, a child might well be able to delve deeper into his or her repertoire of behavioural strategies, and to find more adaptive solutions to interpersonal problems. Thus, we might expect that, other things being equal, young children in particular would exhibit more violent, antisocial behaviour under conditions that are highly stressful, and that they might exhibit more prosocial behaviour in circumstances of greater psychological comfort or security.

Evidence from a variety of sources would seem to be consistent with this view. During the toddler period, one factor that contributes to a child's feelings of psychological comfort is the quality or security of that child's relationship with the mother or other principal caregiver. Thus, it is not surprising that toddlers who have secure relationships with their mothers are found to be more cooperative with their peers and are more likely to initiate positive interaction with unfamiliar adults. A child's emotional state or mood is also an important indicator of psychological comfort, and so it makes sense that children who are rated as happier overall seem to exhibit more prosocial behaviour than those who are not. Similarly, children who are momentarily induced into a positive or happy frame of mind are more likely to behave in prosocial ways than those who are put into negative or sad frames of mind. We can summarize these findings by saying that, as one might expect, conditions of psychological comfort or security seem to facilitate children's production of prosocial behaviour.

In childhood, then, we learn that antisocial behaviour carries a high price, and that, when our capacity for self-regulation is threatened, violence should be our instrument of last resort. The result should be that for older children, as for adults, aggression arises mainly out of insecurity when our capacity for self regulation is threatened most severely and that altruism arises out of security when our capacity for self-regulation seems most assured. There is, of course, little doubt that, in this case, as in so many others, the external conditions of our lives exert substantial influence over our psychological states.

It is important, however, to realise that it is not just external events or conditions in themselves that create psychological states of security or insecurity in us, but also our *interpretations* of these events or conditions. Most of us, for example, will not donate our last dollar to a charitable cause, because we fear that if we do, we may then be unable to satisfy our own basic needs. Some people, however, will and do give their whole wealth to charity. On the other hand, there are also relatively wealthy people who nevertheless remain concerned about their financial security, and do not donate to charities at all. It is not only the objective conditions of wealth or poverty, then, that determine or cause altruistic actions in these cases, or in others like them. It is also the interpretations that we make, which result in the rules that we follow, which in turn generate what prediction of our actions is possible. Thus, in seeking to understand the development of aggression and altruism, we need to concern ourselves not only with a search for objective causes of behaviour, but also with a study of subjective rules of interpretation, and of their applications in action.

4

Developmental Psychology and Genetics

Introduction

Past research consisting of twin and adoption studies has shown that genetic influence is substantial for most domains of developmental psychology. Present research has moved beyond documenting the importance of genetics to investigate the mechanisms by which genetic influences affect behavioural development. The future of genetic research in developmental psychology lies in DNA: Identifying the specific genes responsible for the widespread influence of genetics and using these genes to investigate developmental pathways between genes and behaviour.

The 50th anniversary of the Merrill-Palmer Quarterly provides an occasion to look back on the history of genetic research in developmental psychology and to look forward to its future. This anniversary coincides with the 50th anniversary of the single most important event in the history of genetic research: the discovery of the structure of DNA, which identifies the mechanisms underlying Mendel's laws of inheritance published in 1866.

The brevity of this essay does not permit me to discuss background issues (such as its focus on individual differences within the human species rather than the normative development of our species), to describe methodological issues (such as the twin and adoption methods), or to document thoroughly the research that supports my assertions.

Past

The first attempt to study nature and nurture in the development of behavioural traits was published a year before Mendel's paper. The first twin and adoption studies in developmental psychology were published 80 years ago. Nonetheless, 50 years ago, genetic research was largely ignored by developmental psychologists for three reasons. First, the word genetics became associated with the horrors of Nazi Germany. Second, behaviourism emerged at the same time as the early genetic studies. Behaviourism had a much greater impact on psychology, leading to the dominance of an environmental paradigm, which assumed that we are what we learn. The third reason was that there were relatively few genetics studies until the last 50 years the first textbook on behavioural genetics was only published in 1960, and it focused largely on research with nonhuman animals.

One of the most dramatic shifts in developmental psychology during the past 50 years has been toward acceptance of a more balanced view that recognizes the importance of genetics as well as environment. This shift can be seen in the growing number of genetic papers in mainstream developmental psychology journals and in funded research grants. The public also accepts a major contribution of genetics. For example, a recent poll found that more than 90% of parents and teachers reported that genetics was at least as important as environment for mental illness, personality, learning difficulties, and intelligence.

For nearly every area of psychology that has been studied, twin and adoption studies have shown genetic as well as environmental influence. Genetic research has consistently shown heritable influence in many traditional areas of psychological research, such as psychopathology, personality, cognitive disabilities and abilities, and drug use and abuse. Some areas showing strong genetic influence may be more surprising, such as self-esteem, interests and attitudes, and school achievement. Moreover, the influence of genetic factors is substantial, often accounting for as much as half of the variance.

Consider schizophrenia. Until the 1960s, schizophrenia was thought to be environmental in origin, with theories putting the blame on poor parenting to account for the fact that schizophrenia clearly runs in families. The idea that schizophrenia could run in families for genetic reasons was not seriously considered. Twin and adoption studies changed this view. Twin studies showed that identical twins are much more similar than non identical twins, which suggests genetic influence. If one member of an identical twin pair is schizophrenic, the chances are 45% that the other twin is also schizophrenic. For nonidentical twins, the chances are 17%. Adoption studies showed that the risk of schizophrenia is just as great when children are adopted away from their schizophrenic parents at birth as when children are reared by their schizophrenic parents, which provides dramatic evidence for genetic transmission. There are now intense efforts to identify some of the specific genes responsible for genetic influence on schizophrenia.

In the 1960s when schizophrenia was thought to be caused environmentally, it was important to emphasize the evidence for genetic influence such as the concordance of 45% for identical twins. Now that genetic influence is widely recognized, it is important to emphasize that identical twins are only 45% concordant for schizophrenia, which means that in half of the cases these pairs of genetically identical clones are discordant for schizophrenia. This discordance cannot be explained genetically it must be due to environmental factors. Note that the word environment in genetic research really means nongenetic, which is a much broader definition of environment than is usually encountered in psychology. That is, environment denotes all nonheritable factors, including possible biological events such as prenatal and postnatal illnesses, not just psychosocial factors, The point is that genetics often explains half of the variance of psychological traits, but this means that the other half of the variance is not due to genetic factors. As described in the following section, one of the directions of current genetic research is to investigate environmental influences in genetically sensitive designs in order to understand the interplay between nature and nurture.

Present

Asking whether and how much genetic factors affect psychological dimensions and disorders are important first steps in understanding the origins of individual differences, but these questions are only a beginning. The next steps involve the question "how?" that is, the study of the mechanisms by which genes have their effects. This is the focus of most current genetic research in developmental psychology. Examples include developmental change and continuity, multivariate genetic analysis, and the interplay between genes and environment.

Developmental Change and Continuity. One way in which current genetic research is moving beyond simply demonstrating genetic influence is to ask questions about genetic change and continuity during development. Change in genetic effects from age to age does not necessarily mean that genes are turned on and off during development, although this does happen. Genetic change simply means that genetic effects at one age differ from genetic effects at another age; the same genes could have different effects in the brains of 8-year-olds and 18-year-olds. For example, developmental change in genetic effects is likely to be responsible for the fact that it is difficult to find behavioural markers in childhood for individuals who later become schizophrenic. Although it is possible that "schizophrenia genes" are not turned on until after adolescence, it is more likely that these genes operate the same way before and after adolescence but that they only manifest their hallucinatory and paranoid effects after brain development in adolescence when the brain becomes capable of such highly symbolic processing.

One of the more striking findings of genetic change involves general cognitive ability, often called intelligence and assessed by IQ tests. The magnitude of genetic influence increases steadily from infancy to childhood to adolescence to adulthood. This is surprising because most people would think that environmental factors become increasingly important as experiences accumulate during the life-course. It is not known why the heritability of general cognitive ability increases during development. It is possible that more genes come into play during development, but it also possible that the same genes have greater effects. This latter hypothesis receives support from longitudinal genetic research on age-to-age change and continuity that suggests that the same genes are largely responsible for genetic influence throughout development. If the same genes are involved, how can genetic influence increase? One possibility is genotype-environment correlation, which, as discussed later, refers to correlations between genetic propensities and exposure to experiences. That is, small genetic differences may snowball as we go through life creating environments that are correlated with our genetic propensities.

Multivariate Genetic Analysis. Another important direction for current research is multivariate genetic analysis, which focuses on the covariance (correlation) between traits rather than variance of each trait considered separately. It estimates the extent to which genetic factors that affect one trait also affect another trait. Multivariate genetic research in psychopathology suggests that genetic diagnoses of disorders often differ greatly from traditional diagnoses based on observable symptoms such as anxiety and depression. For example, several studies have shown that the same genes are largely responsible for anxiety and depression. Recent research suggests that this genetic overlap among mental disorders is even broader in that genetic influences yield two broad domains of common psychopathology: internalizing problems that include anxiety, depression, and phobia; and externalizing problems that include antisocial behaviour, conduct disorder, and drug abuse.

Broad effects of genes have also been found in the cognitive domain. Despite the obvious differences between cognitive abilities such as verbal, spatial, and memory abilities, the same genes largely affect all of these cognitive abilities. Genetic overlap is also substantial across learning disabilities such as language, reading, and mathematics disability. Finding such substantial genetic overlap among cognitive abilities and disabilities has far-reaching implications for understanding the brain mechanisms that mediate these genetic effects. Multivariate genetic analysis will also be valuable for investigating genetic overlap between behaviour and biological processes such as hormones, neurotransmitters, and brain imaging. For example, despite the increasing use of cortisol assays in developmental research, genetic research has only recently begun to consider cortisol and its links to behaviour. Similarly, in the cognitive realm, genetic research on neuro imaging measures and their relationship to cognition has just begun.

Interplay Between Genes and Environment. Genetic research is changing the way we think about the environment in development. Two of the most important findings from genetic research involve environmental mechanisms and have come from investigating the environment in genetically sensitive designs. The first finding is that the environment works very differently from the way it has been assumed to work. Instead of making two children growing up in the same family similar to one another, which is what theories of socialization generally assume, genetic research shows that environmental influences that affect behavioural development operate to make children in the same family different. We know this, for example, because genetically unrelated children growing up in the same adoptive family scarcely resemble each other for personality, psychopathology, and cognitive abilities after adolescence. Siblings are similar but for genetic rather than environmental reasons. The environment is important, but environmental influences operate to make children in the same family different, not similar. These environmental influences are called non shared, because they are not shared by children growing up in the same family. Why are children growing up in the same family so different? Although research during the past decade has attempted to identify the specific sources of nonshared environment, only modes progress has been made.

No matter how difficult it may be to find specific non shared environmental factors within the family, it should be emphasized that nonshared environment is generally the way the environment works. Although most research has focused on the family environment, it seems reasonable that experiences outside the family such as experiences with peers and other life events might be richer sources of nonshared environment as children make their own way in the world. It is also possible that chance contribute to nonshared environment in the sense of random noise, idiosyncratic experiences, or the subtle interplay of a concatenation of event. Compounded over time, small differences in experience might lead to large differences in outcome.

The second finding about environmental mechanisms has been called "the nature of nurture". Dozens of twin and adoption studies have shown that when measures of psychological environment (such as parenting, stress, social support) are treated as dependent measures, they show substantial genetic influence. How can this be true, given that environments have no DNA? The answer is that psychological environments can be considered as extended phenotypes of individuals, reflecting genetic differences among individuals as they select, modify, and construct their environments.

Given that environmental as well as behavioural measures show genetic influence, it is reasonable to ask whether associations between environmental measures and behavioural measures are mediated genetically. Multivariate genetic analysis can be used to analyze genetic and environmental contributions to the correlation between environmental measures and behavioural measures. Genetic factors can mediate the correlation between environmental measures and behavioural measure to the extent that the environments respond to genetically influenced characteristics of their children. For example, differences in parenting can be the genetic effect of rather than the environmental cause of children's psychopathology. A general guideline from multivariate genetic research of this sort is that genetic factors are responsible for about half of the phenotypic correlation between measures of the environment and measures of behaviour. For this reason, environmental measures cannot be assumed to be entirely environmental just because they are called environmental measures. A far-reaching implication of this research is that it supports a shift from thinking about passive models of how the environment affects individuals toward models that recognise the active role we play in selecting, modifying, and constructing and reconstructing in memory our experiences.

In summary, genetic research has made some of the most important discoveries about the environment in recent decades, especially about nonshared environment and the role of genetics in experience. More discoveries about environmental mechanisms can be predicted as the environment continues to be investigated in the context of genetically sensitive designs. Much remains to be learned about correlations and interactions between nature and nurture.

Future

The momentum of these findings from current genetic research will carry the field of behavioural genetics well into this new millennium. Twin and adoption studies are called quantitative genetic designs because they can tackle complex traits influenced by multiple genes and multiple environmental factors. The future of genetic research in developmental psychology lies in molecular genetic studies of DNA that will eventually identify specific DNA variants responsible for the widespread influence of genes in psychological development. Identifying these DNA variants will make it possible to address questions about developmental, multivariate, and gene-environment mechanisms with far greater precision and power. For example, in 1993 a gene was identified that increases risk fivefold for dementia later in life. Study of this gene can now be used to investigate its effects earlier in life (developmental), its effect on other types of dementia and other comorbid disorders such as depression (multivariate), and its correlation and interaction with environmental factors, such as its role in worsening the effects of such head injuries as those caused by boxing (gene-environment interplay).

As compared to quantitative genetic studies of twins and adoptees, molecular genetics will have a far greater practical impact on research in developmental psychology because molecular genetic research does not require special populations such as twins or adoptees. In contrast, DNA can be easily and inexpensively obtained (from cheek swabs rather than blood for about $10 per individual) and genotyping of a DNA marker is also inexpensive (about 10 cents per individual). Moreover, devices called gene chips are available that can genotype tens of thousands of genes for an individual in a few hours. Finding genes associated with complex traits is difficult and expensive, but using genes already identified is easy and inexpensive and can add a powerful genetic dimension to any study in developmental psychology.

What has happened in the area of dementia in later life will be played out in many areas of developmental psychology. As mentioned earlier, the only known risk factor for late-onset Alzheimer's disease is a gene, apolipoprotein E, involved in cholesterol transport. A form of the gene called allele 4 increases the risk fivefold for LOAD. Although the association between allele 4 and LOAD was reported only recently, nearly all research on dementia now genotypes participants for apolipoprotein E in order to ascertain whether the results differ for individuals with and without this genetic risk factor. Genotyping apolipoprotein E will also become routine in clinics if this genetic risk factor is found to predict differential response to interventions or treatments. Several developmental psychology studies are currently obtaining DNA on their samples in anticipation of the time when genes are identified that are relevant to their area of interest.

Note that DNA variation has a unique causal status in explaining behaviour. When behaviour is correlated with anything else, the old adage applies that correlation does not imply causation. For example, parenting is correlated with children's behavioural outcomes, but this does not necessarily mean that the parenting causes the outcome environmentally. As mentioned earlier, genetic research has shown that parenting behaviour in part reflects genetic influences on children's behaviour. When it comes to interpreting correlations between biology and behaviour, such correlations are often mistakenly interpreted as if biology causes behaviour. For example, correlations between neurotransmitter physiology and behaviour or between neuro imaging indices of brain activation and behaviour are often interpreted as if brain differences cause behavioural differences. However, these correlations do not necessarily imply causation because behavioural differences can cause brain differences. In contrast, in the case of correlations between DNA variants and behaviour, the behaviour of individuals does not change their genome. Expression of genes changes but the DNA sequence itself does not change. For this reason, correlations between DNA differences and behavioural differences can be interpreted causally: DNA differences cause the behavioural differences but not the other way around.

The single greatest event in the history of genetics was the discovery of the structure of DNA 50 years ago. Understanding the structure of DNA led directly to understanding the two major functions of DNA. The first is the essence of heredity: how DNA reliably duplicates itself by unzipping and dividing the DNA helix up the middle, with each half of the helix re-creating its complement. The second is how DNA codes for proteins, the building blocks of life, although the actual DNA code was not broken for more than a decade after Watson and Crick's paper—the 4-letter alphabet (G, A, T, C nucleotide bases) of DNA is read as 3-letter words that code for the 20 amino acids that are the building blocks of proteins. The crowning glory of the century and a tremendous start to the new century is the Human Genome Project, which in 2001 provided a working draft of the sequence of the 3 billion bases of DNA. However, there is no single human genome: We each have a unique genome because one in a thousand DNA bases, 3 million bases of DNA, vary for at least 1% of the population. Most life scientists are interested in the generalities of the genome, but medical and behavioural scientists are more interested in the variations in the genome that are responsible for hereditary differences. About 2 million of these DNA variants have already been identified and have made it possible to begin to attempt to find some of the genes that affect psychological development, such as the apolipoprotein E gene that is a risk factor for dementia.

Gene identification has been most successful for the thousands of rare single gene disorders in which a mutation in a single gene is necessary and sufficient to cause a disorder. Many of these single-gene disorders have psychological effects for example, more than 200 of these disorders include cognitive effects among their symptoms. However, such single-gene disorders are very rare, with frequencies of .0001 or less. The DNA revolution also provides tools to identify genes responsible for the heritability of common psychological disorders and dimensions. As mentioned earlier, these are usually called complex traits, because they are likely to be influenced by multiple genes as well as by multiple environmental factors. Psychological disorders such as schizophrenia, affective disorders, dementia, autism, reading disability, alcoholism, and hyperactivity are the target of much of this DNA research. Although some genes have been identified for these disorders, the process of identifying genes for complex traits in psychology as well as in medicine has been slower and more difficult than anticipated, probably because complex traits are influenced by many more genes of much smaller effect size than has been assumed.

The most far-reaching ramifications for developmental psychology will come after these genes are identified. Psychology will be central to the new era of genetic research, called the postgenomic era, in which the focus will shift from finding genes to understanding how these genes work. Such postgenomic research is usually considered in relation to the bottom-up strategy of molecular biology, in which a gene's product is identified by its DNA sequence and the function of the gene product is traced through cells and then cell systems and eventually the brain. Psychology lies at the other end of continuum of levels of analysis in the sense that psychology represents an integrationist top-down level of analysis that begins with the behaviour of the whole organism rather than a reductionist bottom-up level of analysis that begins with a single molecule in a single cell. For example, psychologists can ask how the effects of specific genes unfold in behavioural development and how they interact and correlate with experience.

This top-down psychological level of analysis is likely to pay off more quickly in prediction, diagnosis, and intervention, and eventually for behavioural preventions that use genes as early warning systems. Bottom-up and top-down levels of analysis of gene-behaviour pathways will eventually meet in the brain. The grandest implication is that DNA will serve as an integrating force across all of the life sciences, including developmental psychology.

5

Dynamic System for Developmental Theories

Introduction

Dynamic systems views are a completely different sort of theoretical animal than traditional perspectives. The most unusual aspect is the generality of their application. We have come to accept that change such as involved in 'evolution' and 'development' involves genes, and certainly living things, and thus to assume that change in the inanimate world cannot be explained using the same principles. Dynamic systems theorists argue that their theories apply to everything that exists. Consider this argument. As I implied earlier, genes cannot be the source of all evolutionary change as they evolved from something that wasn't genes, but was physical matter. That is, during the process of evolution living things came into being from non-living things. So we know that in order to explain evolution we need a theory in which the principles apply both to the inanimate and animate worlds as they have to include the explanation of the evolution of one from the other. Dynamic theorists do not assume a dichotomy between the principles explaining change for the two sorts of matter, animate and inanimate. On the contrary, their position is that as the principles apply to the interactions of matter, they must apply to both. Of course this does not mean that as humans are intentional organizers and planners of their actions, then so are tornados, for instance. Precisely because humans (and other animals) are designed to be self-promoting, to continue to exist, they have evolved ways of incorporating information about the environments they encounter, unlike the tornado. But it does mean that dynamic systems should be found equally in the functioning of the heart, the atmosphere, snowflakes and psychology.

It shows the now famous pattern that emerges from a mixture of organic and inorganic chemicals studied by Beloussev and Zhabotinsky in the 1950s and 1960s, and now named the BZ reaction, in which, to simplify, bromous acid is produced. It looks like this because a cycle of interaction keeps repeating itself. Involves the same chemical interaction? No, it is not a chemical reaction at all, but shows the changes that occur when individual amoebas, which themselves developed form germinated spores, start to move and join together as they do as part of the developmental cycle of the slime mould, Dicyostelium discoideum. Similar patterns are found elsewhere in nature. They look the same because the dynamics of their production is the same. Goodwin explains:

> These examples show that what counts in the production of spatial patterns is not the nature of the molecules and other components involved, such as cells, but the way these interact with one another in time (their kinetics) and space (their relational order): how the state of one region depends upon the state of neighbouring regions). These two properties together define the behaviour of a dynamic system.

Dynamic models are thus especially useful because the properties of dynamic processes are independent of the mechanics of the process, an oscillation is an oscillation whether it is a spring, a pendulum or a joint in motion. Thus the descriptions it offers can apply to all sorts of behaviour of all sorts of systems, like the development of bromous acid, an amoeba, a snowflake, a thunderstorm, walking or facility with calculus.

In addition, organismic development is an open system: it exchanges energy and matter with its environment. This property is crucial for two reasons. First, if the organism were a closed system the second law of thermodynamics would hold, and the energy in the system, the organism, would dissipate, so there would be no differentiated structure, just as ice, a result of the 'development', the self-organisation of water between 0 and -4 degrees, is the same all over. Organisms can confound this principle only by reorganising internally to become more effectively coupled to the environment, more differentiated. And this is the second property. This process of internal reorganisation is the means whereby the organism becomes more differentiated, as it develops structures which couple it adaptively to the ecology. Indeed, that is what development is. This coupling, like evolving a skeleton to cope with gravity, or means of navigation based upon complex invariances in the movement of stars, or the sun, or learning a language, both constrains the ways in which interactions between the organism and environment can take place and afford others.

Thirdly, because dynamic models focus on change over time they are better equipped for the analysis of process, of how change occurs, a matter we will look into in more detail in a separate section. So as all dynamic systems have these characteristic properties, we can apply what has already been found about the properties of such systems to the study of human development. We can thereby move away from the sterile focus on stages, to transitions, the dynamics of change.

Another obvious feature of these views lies in the unit of analysis used. It is assumed that the behaviour and function of any object, organism or phenomenon can be understood only in relation to the system of which it is a part. Systems have multiple components, so it is never assumed that any single preformed cause will determine outcomes. Rather, outcomes depend upon the particular pattern of interactions between the components, the factors. This is exactly the position we have reached both from the arguments and the above point regarding the evolution of life itself; that there can be no dichotomy between organism and environment, the unit of analysis must be the system. Further, it implies that the functional relations between sub-systems is close, so that for the case of psychological development this means there must be both a close coupling between the perceptual, action and cognitive sub-systems of the organism and between these sub-systems and the characteristics of the environment and relations between them, just as we have been arguing.

A Different View of Causality

Because these theories start from different premises their assumptions about change will be different. The tradition in psychology is to look for linear relations, where the greater the amount of a relevant variable, the greater the effect. The reason for this tradition is the lack of belief in interaction as a force for change: it is assumed that causal impetus is limited to a preformed entity. But the nature of the relationship between sub-systems in a biological system is non-linear and the same applies to all dynamic systems: one cannot predict how the whole system will behave just by knowing the values of the inputs to it. A change in one aspect of one internal subsystem, e.g. in physiology, could make some difference, or none at all. The same is true for a change in an external environmental variable. It is often the case that a small change in conditions can lead to a massive reorganisation of the behaviour of the system, non-linear and unpredictable change. The reason that this is the case is that it is internal reorganisation that determines change, and changes in input are just one factor that can affect that. This process is called a phase-shift. And what follows from this interactivity and non-linearity is that the nature of the changes which do occur depend upon the interactions that occur, not being fixed by any particular value of any one variable, as in the traditional independent variable. The analysis of such forms of change requires a different mathematics than we are used to, it requires nonlinear techniques. There are a variety of these, beyond the scope of this book, and the scope of my knowledge, but as an example, catastrophe theory provides the mathematics to describe the different forms of abrupt change observed in systems, and chaos theory describes changes which are not at all random, being describable exactly by differential equations, but which can look random as small changes to conditions often 'precipitate' a variety of new and different behaviours.

What is involved here is a different idea of causality. On the traditional model a significant difference in behaviour would be taken to imply a significant difference in the value or type of independent variables, because change is presumed to be linear rate of change of behaviour is proportional to rate of change of independent variable. Without that assumption we are not forced to assume that conditions have changed significantly if behaviour has, nor that conditions have not changed if behaviour has not. There is a relation between the various causal factors and behavioural outcomes, but because it is from complex interactions between the components that change arises, where a small change can lead to a complex reorganisation of the system, the relation is not linear.

This means that the whole approach to science is different. The traditional method of experimentation which assumes the linear relation between changes in independent and dependent variable, underpins the controlled experiment, where all variables are fixed except the independent one. One of the reasons for this methodology would have been the lack of a mathematical means of dealing with the behaviour of multiple complex interactions in systems. But in addition, people, especially the scientists themselves, came to consider the method to be the right and only proper way to do science. Such a procedure needs to be recognised as based upon a set of assumptions. It assumes linearity, a very similar assumption to the gradualism assumed in evolution, as it always expects that there cannot be catastrophic jumps in outcomes, that there can be no build up of dynamic energy which must be released, that various small internal changes will not eventually be followed by major reorganisation. It assumes that there is not a complex of factors which has its own unique composition so that the result of the interaction of all the component factors can always surprise us. The more we actually observe what happens in development the more we see that such assumptions are simply not justified.

The behaviour of organisms and inanimate processes is characterized by two, opposite sorts of situation. We observe flux, sudden change, but we also observe periods of stability, called attractor states. The persistence is named the stability of the system and the adjustment to changing internal and external conditions its adaptability. We hear of and are not surprised by dramatic and apparently chaotic fluctuations in many aspects of life, whether it be the populations of particular species, changes in the weather, changes in our mind, for that matter. There is messiness, yet there is order. These same characteristics become ever more evident in studies of the development of organisms, including humans. Dynamic systems theories are the only theories that assume this combination of order and apparent (but not real) disorder and predict it. When there is order it looks as if the components of the system co-operated to produce it, or that the system selected it, was attracted to it. The set of factors comes to appear to act as one. Moreover, this pattern will persist even though the inputs to the system vary. The process by which it arrives is called 'self-organisation'. However, just as typically, it is found that points are reached where variation to the input leads to fluctuations. These are points at which the dynamic equilibrium is disturbed, a variety of sorts of transitory behaviours, sorts of warnings of massive change, occur, and soon a new stability does indeed arise from another self-organisation.

Focusing on Human Development

Self-organization

Because there is no external programme or fixed, internal regulator, any increasing complexity and differentiation results from spontaneous, internal rearrangement, known as self-organisation. It is the process by which internal relations realign themselves in an attempt to optimize the relations between the organism and the environment. It is, as I now argue, the alternative to preformation.

We observe order as well as disorder in development. We thus have to account for it. The relative stability and simplicity of many developmental outcomes has lent weight to the interpretation that it is the effect of a relatively stable and simple cause, a preformed programme. As we have already seen, no such conclusion is justified. The common interactionist explanation is that genetic and environmental factors combine in some way. But why should combination lead to order? If there is no need for self-organization in dynamic systems, and as I say, most do not yet subscribe to the view that there is, then the interactions they refer to should lead to behaviours which are a mixture of (organised) genetically controlled behaviour and (organised) experience controlled behaviour. But why should the mixture resulting from the interaction be organised? What organises it? Preformationism cannot do the job, as it is not about interaction. Ordinary 'interactionism' cannot, because it is not dynamic, non-linear systems theory. Only dynamic systems theory explicitly places the organization of the system itself, from within, as a major and ubiquitous feature of all developmental change.

The self-organisation can involve reorganization of internal, biomechanical structures, itself a complex of sub-sub systems, as when a new form of locomotion emerges. It can involve a reorganisation of the internal psychological structures, as when knowledge of aspects of language emerge. It can involve a reorganisation of the relations between the external and internal factors, as when a child 'takes over' more of the task demands after scaffolding has helped their development on a given task. It can involve a reorganisation of the timing of a behaviour contingent on an external factor, amount of clothing worn, as in the case when Bensen, reported in Ulrich, showed that babies born in the winter and spring in an area where seasonal variations were large, crawled three weeks earlier than those born in the summer and autumn. The early crawlers had had more experience of crawling because they were in less restrictive clothing, because the weather had warmed up at a time when experience would make a difference.

Despite the huge complexity of interacting factors, we do find that generic forms of behaviour do emerge, are selected by the process of self-organisation. Infants do tend to crawl before they walk. They do tend to produce certain sounds before others. They do get from lying to sitting by pushing their trunk upward, leaning slightly to one side and bringing legs forward, by flexing their knee and hip joints. And despite the tendency for generic self-organisation we will come across cases where a small change in conditions can change the way this occurs. Infants with Down's syndrome, who have a greater range of hip motion, just one tiny part of the internal, bodily sub-system, get to the sitting position a different way, as they can bring each leg forward on either side of the body. All these are instances of self-organisation.

Collective Variables (Order Parameters)

The characteristic behaviours of the self-organised system are said to be due to what is called the collective variable or order parameter, that regularity, often describable by a single mathematical equation, which shows the collective properties of the system under different conditions. The linear equivalent would be the dependent variable, but the difference here is that it describes the reasonably simple outcome, the 'collective dynamics' of numerous complex interactions. The order parameter is seen as typically ensuring that the sub-systems involved maintain their states so that the interactive flux remains the same, the condition for the regularity being maintained. That is to say, it looks as if it keeps them in order, ensuring that the various subsystems do not 'upset' the overall order. This is not the same as saying that the collective variable causes the behaviour, because that variable is effective only when a given pattern of factors constitutes the causal flux.

Control Parameters

Even though a vast number of factors have been involved in the interactions from which the collective order emerged (the collective variable, order parameter again), it is often the case that a small number (sometimes one) of variables or relations are particularly relevant in affecting the collective variable. These are called control parameters. It is these which are of most significance in holding the system in stability, constraining the effects of any other variation on the system. But they are also of equal significance in that when they reach a critical value or boundary condition they trigger reorganization and a phase-shift occurs. Control parameters are thus important both in maintaining stability and in evoking change.

No assumption of continued influence can be made for such variables. For instance, at birth infants produce stepping patterns if held in upright posture. These are lost when the infant is about two months old. It was thought that this was due to 'maturation'. What control parameter is responsible for this change? Thelen and Fisher found that the rapid weight gain of human infants in the first two or three months was mainly due to fat deposition, and the loss of the stepping ability in an upright posture was probably due to a drop in the power to weight ratio. That is, this was the control parameter, that variable in which variation at critical levels is associated with a phase-shift, a sudden transition in the order parameter.

When older this will not normally be a control parameter. Similar parameters may control the transition from crawling to walking. Ronnqvist and Hopkins found that newborns may, contrary to general belief, be able to attain and maintain a midline head position, but do not normally do so because their neck muscles are not strong enough to overcome the powerful effects of gravity on the head. In this case the control parameter may be neck muscle power. Clearly, it only has this function early in development.

Here are some more examples of different control parameters. The energy applied by a horse in motion is a control parameter. As the energy increases it moves through successive boundary conditions which correspond to the abrupt transitions from trot to canter to gallop (each of which is defined by dynamic, mathematical equations relating to the phase relationships between limb movements, as is the case for all movements of all organisms with legs). When a rider 'drives' the horse on, they become the control parameter. The ratio of size and shape of fingers to size of object to be grasped has been shown to be another control parameter in motor development, affecting the order parameter, the grip pattern observed. An example from cognitive development comes from van der Maas and Hopkins, who observed that short-term memory and 'field dependency' are two control parameters affecting performance on a conservation task. In the field of social psychology Dunbar found that as group size increased there was a change in the manner in which social cohesion developed. Thus group size was the control parameter. Since 1960 it has been known that infants would use the invariances which specify a 'cliff edge' (i.e. specify a sudden increase in depth of surface supporting self), to know what was there and to respond adaptively by avoiding it. It has also been regularly found that there are large individual differences between infants in their tendency to avoid the edge. It appears likely that differences in prefrontal lobe development, which controls inhibition of motor activity, underlies the difference and are therefore acting as one of the control parameters. It is as well to remember that in all these examples there is no fixed plan, no preformation. The controls work in some situations and become irrelevant in others.

There are three sorts of constraints, as Newell pointed out, which can act as control parameters, organismic, environmental or task-specific. For instance, the strength of muscles, an organismic factor, sets limits on what actions can be performed, as does the oxygen level in the blood; the carrying out of a task in water, an environmental constraint, will alter performance, as could being able to use a tool; learning to communicate depends upon task-specific contingent responses from another, while sorting a pack of cards, by suit, would involve and require different abilities, like dexterity, again task-specific.

A control parameter has very different properties from an independent variable and without the benefit of its appropriation from dynamic systems views, I rather doubt if its significance in development would be appreciated. We would not be looking for variables which have this amazing mix of qualities, being dependent upon the rest of the interactive flux in so far as they operate only for given patterns of that flux; constraining change up to a boundary condition; effecting change when they reach that point, and furthermore, ceasing to be relevant at a later point in the emerging developmental system, when the interactive flux has changed again. It is part of the dialectical character of systems change and once we appreciate this we can accept the fluidity, the dynamism involved in interactive effects. With the benefit of knowledge of its role from other systems it has been possible to see something of its potential role in human development. And it is very early days yet. To make real progress using dynamic systems theory it will be necessary to identify different control parameters for different conditions, and to identify those conditions, rather than simply to argue that a complex of interacting factors is jointly responsible. But you must understand that without such a recognition of the relevance of dynamic systems views to human development, we would not even be able to identify the relevant questions. Such views are important for this reason alone.

Control Parameters and the Production Levels of Knowledge

Those that are species-specific control parameters, like the extent to which a human arm muscle can flex and extend, or the range of movement of a joint, or maximum and minimum levels of oxygen in the blood compatible with life, constrain development in generic ways, but do not specify exactly what actions or thoughts will be selected. They have generic effects in that they set boundary conditions. Individual or task-specific control parameters, like aerobic efficiency, will have more specific effects, but still, of course, within the species-specific boundary conditions. So what, you may ask. The matter becomes significant when this argument is applied to the development of knowledge. The questions become: what are the generic, speciesspecific constraints on information extraction? How do these relate to specific learning, or selection by experience? In dynamic systems terms, what are the control parameters for knowledge production, both species-specific and individual, and how do these systematically relate to each other?

Types of Attractors

An attractor is a stable state, like walking, or reaching and grasping accurately. It represents a solution to a problem of how to achieve something. There are four sorts of attractors. The first is called a fixed-point attractor, and refers to the existence of a single, stable equilibrium point, like the end-point of a reach or a grasp, where action consists in a trajectory (the reach) terminating at a point (location of object) and an accurate form is roughly the same for everyone, there not being alternative stable forms. At first there would be errors in reaching too far, and not far enough, and both of these would reduce over time till the error was minimal. The meeting of the axes corresponds to zero error in any direction, so the circular trajectory, gradually homing in on zero, corresponds to the decreasing error in reaches, over time, anywhere about the point to be reached. It also exactly describes the motion of a real pendulum swinging past the vertical, but gradually reducing in amplitude, because the dynamics are identical. Similarly, the dynamics of the control of the various muscles and joints is exactly the same for an arm as for a spring, involving flexion of the various muscles at various times, in relation to each other, and variation in the angles between limbs at joints. In both, account has to be taken of inertia, a property of all dynamic systems, and the laws of force, mass and acceleration have to be obeyed, because the arm is matter as well, and thus subject to its laws.

The second sort of attractor is a limit cycle or periodic attractor, where a continuous oscillation with a fixed amplitude and frequency occurs. Walking, in which various oscillations of parts of the body occur, which are repeated with each stride, is one case. Amplitude (from top of peak to bottom of trough) is length of stride and time for a stride is the time, on the horizontal axis, between peaks. Hence you will be able to work out that the person has a stride which is exactly half as long as the other, but that they stride twice as often (so, as it happens, a graph of velocity alone would be identical). Third we have quasiperiodic or taurus attractors. These arise when two attractors are both having an influence, but neither is dominant. The pattern of activity in non-nutritive sucking in the neonate is described by such an attractor, based upon the interaction of sucking and swallowing factors. Finally we have the chaotic or strange attractor.

Changes at Transitions

Wimmers describe how catastrophe theory can help in understanding the development of action and Hartelman, van der Maas and Molenaar discuss the criteria for transitions. When change is imminent, dynamic systems show the signs. Catastrophe theory specifies the various conditions which can be met when a phase-shift is going to occur. If human development is describable by this particular dynamic systems theory, we should be able to observe the same sorts of conditions occurring in human behaviour.

Gilmore identified eight criteria, or flags, as evidence for the existence of transitions. All of them must involve a sudden change in behaviour, taking the form of a jump of some sort, like divergence, when two similar trends diverge widely, or an increase in variability of a behaviour, a greater sensitivity to perturbation near a transition, or a slowing down of the system in returning to its stable state after perturbation, regressions, etc.

A wonderful example of transition and speed of change at a phase-shift is seen in certain weather conditions we have all observed. Differences in air density lead to hailstones being formed, with the smaller, lighter hailstones moving to the top of the growing cloud, forming 'the anvil' shape and the bigger, heavier ones not being able to rise so much and being held in the main body of the cloud. As the stones pass each other the lighter become negatively charged and the heavier positively charged. Over time the forces of repulsion grow bigger and bigger. Then, with no change in rate of action, the system collapses, huge amounts of electrical and sound energy are released, until the system reorganises into a new stability. The phase-shift, the self-organisation, is called a thunderstorm, and the energy release is thunder and lightening. Ulrich provides another example, less familiar in Britain. When there is a sufficient temperature difference between the earth and the atmosphere, and the pressure and humidity are within certain limits, 'the collective interplay of multiple factors results in the emergence of a distinctly recognisable pattern, a funnel cloud'. As Ulrich points out, no one feels the need to posit any preformed instructions, any 'plans of action', to account for these events. We accept both that novel outcomes emerge, novel in the sense that the cloud did not exist a few minutes before, and that this is the sort of thing that happens in weather systems, that 'recognisable', stable forms emerge, like funnel clouds, that huge changes do occur, and that these are marked by predictable 'flags'.

Some of this, certainly the terminology, may sound disconnected with your ordinary experience. We all already understand at a common sense level how pervasive dynamic non-linear transitions are. In normal conversation it is quite in order to refer to changes of heart, to violent changes of mood, to sudden rows, to inexplicable and uncontrollable changes in our mental states or physical states. We do not have difficulty with the notion of 'the last straw', just a simple example of non-linear change as it is the tiniest change the last straw which leads to the large change. We all know and accept that as water goes through temperature changes it changes qualitatively in form, from water to ice, and can just as easily vapourize at a given point. We know, using another example from Thelen and Smith, that we take utterly for granted the abrupt locomotory phase-shifts that characterize the changes between different gaits of a horse as it walks (one attractor state), then shifts abruptly (a phase-shift) to a trot, a qualitatively different mode of locomotion, then a canter, then a gallop. The gait is the collective variable, the phenomenon which shows the collective properties of the system, under different conditions. Energy applied is the control parameter. It looks as if locomotion is under very simple control, because the attractor states observed are simple. This is a mirage, due to the self-organizing properties of this particular dynamic system in action. By the way, here is an experiment for the future. Take one horse. Place on moon. Observe how self-organisational processes affected its emergent modes of locomotion in the same reduced gravity that radically altered human locomotion.

We accept dynamic systems change in our non-academic lives even if we do not use the associated language. We know that when two friends tark to each other before they talk to you it can make a difference, but we do not normally call it the complex interaction of external factors. We know that anxiety at a nervous eye-twitch (the anxiety being both a cause and an effect of the anxiety) can make your neck ache, but do not normally call it the interaction of internal factors. We know that you can end up behaving very nervously and your friend reacts to this, but do not normally call this the interaction of external with internal factors. And we know that a stable state may arise from this mix, or a huge change may take place. However, another dichotomy we have been brought up with, theoretical/practical, induces those of us not concerned with theory to regard our knowledge as inferior, so our common sense knowledge of dynamic interactions is not accorded the validity it should be, not even by ourselves.

How is Skilled Action Possible?

One of the important advances in dynamic systems came from the work of Bernstein, who was the first to point out that all behaviour appears to involve setting the values of so many variables that it looks, on the face of it, as if even simple action is impossible. As Hopkins and Butterworth describe, the human body has nearly 800 muscles, 200 bones and more than 100 joints. Every one of these is always in a given position in relation to all the others, and has a certain velocity. This musculoskeletal system can only operate because of the links to the nervous system, which involves 10^{14} neurons and 10^3 varieties of nerve cell. Walking directly involves 3 joints and over 50 muscles in each leg, but also involves setting and varying the action of various other muscles and joints which are less directly involved but still need organising if we are not to fall over. All this assumes no variation in external context, an ideal which is not encountered. It seems absolutely impossible that the execution of action could be organized by the brain separately controlling every single one of these components, including the effects of their interactions. Nor could a preformed, central, executive plan take account of all this vast complexity, interaction and accommodation to varying conditions. There has to be a way of simplifying the problem.

Bernstein argued that the only way it could be achieved was by constraining the action of a whole group of muscles at once so that they were set at certain amounts of tension, not allowed to vary, and thus could be 'forgotten' about. We can in fact see this happening in the development of, for instance, leg movements. Thelen described how the leg joints are kept fixed in the initial kicking that babies exhibit in the first week of life, an obvious form of constraint for one of the many movement sub-systems. Later, between one and five months they relax the fix and kicking is practised while the joints allow the attached feet, lower legs and upper legs to vary with respect to each other (under the evolved constraints of the human body). At about six months, the more controlled organisation of these joints is reassembled, this time with the capacity to use the limbs for crawling. Bernstein argued that at first the 'freezing' of the relations between some groups of muscles or joints takes place which simplifies the complex problem of motor control by not having to take account of some possible variations. The infant explores this constrained system, seeing what can be done within it, realizing its opportunities for action, its affordances. It finds out what actions and effects it can have. The constraints lead to affordances. Once there has been sufficient experience with this arrangement, the restriction is released and the movement sub-system can be reorganised. Exploration of this arrangement then begins, and so on. Of course this applies to many coordinative structures, as these sub-systems are called. As a result, 'impossibly' complex acts are possible, based upon the initial restriction of possible variations through organized constraint at a sub-system level.

Dynamic Systems and Development

We can describe the process of the development of leg movements in terms of my central hypothesis. As the infant of less than one month explores a particular configuration of restraints to reveal what it can do, it is effectively exploring a task-space. Initially the 'space' is highly constrained in the sense that the task is simple, as not much can be varied. But so is the behaviour, as skill is limited. The task and the exploration and the information produced are thus all relatively undifferentiated. Then that particular set of constraints can be relaxed and exploration about how to control parts of the body in a new, looser and thus slightly more complex and differentiated arrangement can begin, but only because of the information gained in the previous phase. The infant only learns to crawl because it learned to kick, etc. This information then gets used to aid the next form of constraints, of self-organisation, and so on.

A surface behavioural pattern exists, which appears as stability, transitions and phase-shifts, but underlying each period of 'stability' is dynamic exploration of a given arrangement. The exploration of the initial, constrained task-space produces undifferentiated information, which is then used to inform self-organization into a more complex set of constraints which affords more complex exploration and produces more differentiated information. This is exactly the same as we have already suggested as our main principle for the production of knowledge, and it is completely different to saying that the system is preformed, because each stability enables new, different interactions and it is only from these that new developmental products emerge. The developmental system can thus be construed as the process of successive constraint and release of system variables so that the affordances of each system can be explored. Though it is not emphasized in the theory, change which has this character, where reaching a stable state is also to reach a set of conditions from which change will inevitably emerge in both components and their products because of their mutual interactivity, is the core of dialectical theory. Development is just that complex of interaction over time, between the organism and environment by which these processes and products emerge and dissolve.

There may be some confusion over the fact that I have suggested that dynamic systems cover both biological and non-biological processes. That does not mean there are not special sorts of questions that biologists ask. To make clear that I am not distancing myself from a biological perspective I will set out now how I perceive the relation between what is biological and what is the subject of a dynamic systems perspective. In the first place, biological explanations of behaviour, because they are explanations, must specify the necessary and sufficient factors involved for the behaviour to occur. In systems terms the relevant factors and the role of control parameters in the development of attractors and phase-shifts in behaviour need to be identified and the manner of their interaction revealed. In the second place, because the specifically biological assumption is made that organisms behave in the way they do because it has a function for them in the contexts they typically inhabit, it becomes necessary to locate the functions of behaviour within their phylogenetic and ontogenetic contexts, that is, systems. This is a long-standing emphasis in ethology, but should become a new and crucial one in psychology, as some have argued already.

I think a clarification of what the typical contexts for humans are and have been will clarify what 'biological' means. First, it is impossible to ignore the evolutionary context, so questions of evolutionary fitness are relevant. Bodies and behaviours represent the history of a species. Humans really do have arms, birds do have beaks, etc. and this has a significant effect upon what they can now do. This applies both to explanations of the immediate value of an act, such as the clearing of an area around the nest that results from picking up the shell pieces and depositing them elsewhere and the long-term fitness of this tidying-up process in aiding survival chances of offspring. It is equally impossible to ignore the ontogenetic context, as behaviour must be sensitive, as we have seen, to idiosyncratic contingencies.

The immediate function and the evolutionary value of behaviour are both about coupling. Both sorts of coupling fit action to its context, so coupling through learning or coupling by evolution are equally biological. History is represented, whether the history is five minutes or 5 million years old. It also obviously follows that what is learned cannot determine whether it is to be counted as biological or not, only its function can. Thus, caretaking, bus catching and reading are all just as much parts of our biological environment as food and drink. In all cases coupling involves the selection of changes which provide a better fit between the physical and psychological form and functions of the organism and those of the environment. All such changes and all such processes are biological. But the forms of change, and the relations between organismic change and the contextual conditions, both follow laws which describe a wide variety of natural systems. Development is thus the change in dynamic, biological systems by which a coordination of the organism and environment occurs. Biological accounts must include all sorts of adaptation to all sorts of structure, invariance, whether these be of food distribution, prey habits, fashion fads, social norms or language rules, whatever. The model is thus explicitly ecological in character and is generic in applying to all ancestral and present forms of invariant, environmental structure and levels of them, between the humans and those environments and within the humans.

The accounts must include all sorts of adaptation to all sorts of structure, invariance, whether these be of food distribution, prey habits, fashion fads, social norms or language rules, whatever. The model is thus explicitly ecological in character and is generic in applying to all ancestral and present forms of invariant, environmental structure and levels of them, between the humans and those environments and within the humans.

But I am not being clear about what it is that travels in these dynamic systems. What is used? What is transformed? To move towards an answer I now have to introduce you more thoroughly to the ecological psychology of J.J. Gibson.

6

Ecological, Dynamic Systems for Human Thinking

Introduction

One involves an important attempt to dispense with the nature/nurture dichotomy, but it is particularly instructive because we can identify, even within the attempts to change, the forces of traditional thinking restraining the attempt. I hope to clarify both the old and more importantly the new ways of thinking by emphasizing the failure as well as the success of the attempt.

The other two involve contrasting computational metaphors of human thinking and change. One you will be familiar with, to the extent you may not realize it is only a metaphor: the mind as serial computer. The other is a connectionist model, a simple robot in which 'perception', 'cognition' and 'action' are closely coupled. I describe them to show how the different assumptions about dichotomies between perception, cognition and action, between complex mind and simple body, make all the difference to what 'psychology' can be demonstrated by these computers. The aims are again the same, to highlight the way in which assumptions control our thinking, and how different assumptions lead to very different outcomes.

But to prepare the way, some further analysis of ecological and traditional thinking. If the traditional position were valid, we would not find cases where a developmental outcome or behaviour was not attributable to either form of cause. But when the man walked on the moon, or rather, didn't, the assumption that walking was due to 'nature' was violated. But nor was the change in preferred means of locomotion the result of learning. Neither of the traditional explanations work. But they are supposed to form not just exclusive categories, but an exhaustive category system; no other form of explanation is possible. The traditional position cannot be correct. But there is a form of explanation which does account for the observation. We encountered it already when considering the properties of internal, organismic structure and of external, environmental structure. This section is critical.

I observed that genes and indeed many internal products are a universal and necessary part of internal structure for every species, that they display properties both of stability and of change, but that for developmental change to occur requires that exactly the same properties are displayed by the developmentally relevant external conditions with which the internal ones are in interaction. Development thus depends upon the interactions between two sorts of contexts, one internal to the skin and one external to it. At every moment it is in the interactions between and within these two contexts that change occurs and thoughts and actions are selected. Both are necessary for development but only their joint occurrence over the period of the selection of adaptations is sufficient for the change to get established. If and only if the components cooccur can the interactions reliably occur and a system of developmental products reliably emerge. The two contexts in interaction form one system, the developmental system.

It briefly consider factors involved in migration and we will see that external factors, like the movement of the stars, and the changing light/dark cycles, and internal factors, like hormonal changes and muscle development, are just a few of the many influences in the interacting complex from which the adaptive action of migration, to the right place at the right time, emerges. When humans walk and how, emerges from the complex interaction of the biodynamics of the body which enables some actions, like arm flexion and alternate leg movement, and prohibits others, like flying, from the external structures and forces, air containing oxygen, gravity, surrounding fluid (gas or liquid) which may afford swimming in but not walking on, and from the psychological structures, motives, intentions, fears, etc. which affect what we would try to do, be scared of, feel obliged in respect of, etc. Which aspects are relevant for a given situation depend upon the relation of organism, context and task at any given moment. If walking up a hill is the task, a change in terrain, mud (increased deformability of surface), altitude, attitude are a few of the many factors involved.

Thus the organisation of our bodies affords (makes possible) actions of certain sorts but not of others, as a result of phylogeny, and the organisation of the environment affords certain actions or uses but prohibits others. However, the form of influence of each does not act separately of the other. In fact the opposite is true. What the body can or cannot do is totally relative to the conditions, the environment encountered and what the environment affords or constrains depends upon which species or individual we are referring to. Humans can run, but when we say this we are stating a shorthand for 'run if there is a sufficiently rigid surface, oxygen is reliably encountered, etc.', conditions which can change. When attempting to describe the affordances of the external structure the same applies they mean nothing till we specify the organism as well. The affordances and constraints of a mountain hillside in Rwanda are very different for me than for a gorilla, and even more different for a conifer, or a human infant on their own. The dynamic structure, the organisation of the external environment matters, but for understanding and explaining development it is the *relation* of that dynamic structure to the internal dynamic structure that determines developmental and behavioural outcomes. And it cannot matter how long the structure took to develop (talons, brains), only what its characteristics are in relation to those of the environment. Thus the interaction of a structure that just came into being two seconds ago, like my foot on this piece of earth, with one that has been around for a hundred million years is a common event. It does not matter if one was selected in evolutionary time and one in a moment, all that matters is the relation between two interacting structures.

Further, what we can and cannot do with an environment is as much to do with psychological factors as internal or external physical ones. These affect what we perceive what you 'see' depends upon what you need or what you know, and they hugely influence what you think, remember, understand, value, plan thereby what you may do. Put all three sorts of factors together and we have the following scenario: a human organism which is a specific physical realization, having legs, fingers, joints of various sorts, plus a level of fitness, fatigue, etc., operating in a specific physical ecology which both enables and constrains actions of different sorts, with specific psychological resources and impediments which equally both enable and constrain what thoughts and actions can be chosen. Each of these is meaningless except in relation to the other two. Thus every act we ever carry out occurs only as the complex outcome of interactions between all these sorts of factors. And each of these has a phylogeny and an ontogeny.

In the Introduction we saw that a change in the value of one variable was indeed sufficient to dramatically alter the outcome from the whole pattern of influence: walking was replaced by jumping as the more efficient, preferred mode of locomotion for that internal/psychological/external set or system of affordances and constraints, for the total pattern of forces in interaction at that time for that individual. It was not replaced because of a bodily reason or factor, or a psychological reason or an environmental reason. Nor could it ever be. It was replaced because the overall pattern settled into a different state, self-organized differently. It becomes irrelevant to the ascription of causal power to try to place the origin of the outcome in one part of the causal flux or another. It is only from the whole pattern of forces and constraints that the most efficient pattern of action emerges. This is self-organisation.

The organism/environment dichotomy makes no sense in this world. The inner/outer dichotomy is no help. The biological/learning/social offers nothing. All any of these dichotomies does is to try to break apart what is a unity, to artificially categorize the world. It is the total pattern which matters. Change that pattern, that set of relations, and the action, the functioning of the organism is itself likely to change.

Types of Interaction and the Integration of Nature and Nurture Revisited

When a young gull pecks at the spot on the beak of the parent herring gull the adult regurgitates food. It is typical for the adults to have the spot, typical for the young to see it, to need food, and to have internal brain structures which interact with the visual input from the spot to lead to pecking at it. This little dynamic, self-organising system involves species-typical components, of which some are part of the external context and some part of the internal context, in interaction, and has evolved to generally ensure the chick gets food. It 'knows' how to do this in the sense that it does not require practice at specific beaks to learn it. But the beak that was pecked at was a unique beak, and so was the beak pecking it. And of course they were bound to be. There aren't any other sorts of beaks in the material world. These species-typical interactions are thus also necessarily acts of individuals and thereby affected by the individuals characteristics, their particular shape, size, strength, vision, but also their learning, of how to move, given the young gulls relatively weak muscles, of when, given their appetite. Similarly, the gull will be learning various things, which involves interactions between specifics in the external context leading to changes in internal contexts, brain organisation. But these changes are totally constrained by what learning and what behaviour is possible for the species. There are separate sorts of interactions, ontogenetic and phylogenetic, in theory, but all necessarily involve the other sort in practice.

Remember the caddis fly that has the evolved capacity to build its own extended phenotype. The larvae typically locate, pick up and manipulate individual stones during their unique life, stones which may not have existed when the extended phenotype first evolved. But the action of the caddis must be tailored to the exact position and weight of individual stones, fitting their species-typical action exactly to the unique contexts they are encountering. The construction of this extended phenotype thus only emerges from the combination of knowledge afforded by species-typical interactions, knowledge of action in the species-typical context, and knowledge afforded by individual interactions between the individual larvae and the individual contexts they encounter, knowledge of size, location, and adaptive action in respect of the individual stones under analysis. That stones have locations and extension is species-typical, but the particular locations and size are not. Production of the adaptive phenotype is dependent upon using both sorts of knowledge together. As we will see, this ability for systems to arise in which products of interactions over phylogenetic time and those in ontogenetic time are integrated together is of great import for the evolution of developmental systems.

These are not special cases. Behavioural outcomes will always be a function of phylogenetic (contingent interactions which have been selected over evolutionary time) factors and ontogenetic factors (contingent interactions selected during an individual lifetime). It is impossible for an individual organism not to be operating within its phylogenetic context. But it is equally impossible for a species to change in any other way than through and in the individual lives in individual contexts of individual members of the species.

Selection of Cognition and Action Ignores the Origin or Location of Factors

Again, however long these interactions have been going on, irrespective of whether they arose over evolutionary or ontogenetic time, the outcomes depend upon the contingent presence and thereby interaction of the relevant components, like beaks and visual input and brains. For instance, cognitive impairment to the herring gull chick, a contingent state, can immediately stop the species-typical interaction of internal and external structure required for the peck to occur, however long that adaptation had taken to evolve. The loss of the (contingent) value of gravity species-typically encountered on earth immediately led to the start of a self-organisation of locomotion. In this case (and in all others) it matters not one iota that the physical structure of the human body has taken evolutionary time to develop and has done so in ways heavily constrained by the invariant force of gravity on earth, etc., while the contingent interaction of a human body trying to get around on a surface which afforded walking but with a changed force of gravity for the first time in the history of that species (apart from simulation), had only just occurred seconds before. The phylogenetic context and the immediate gravitational context interacted and produced a novel outcome for the history of the species.

Selected in Natural Selection

Darwinian explanations of adaptations did not specify the precise circumstances, the specific context in which a behavioural phenotype would be adaptive. They would identify some general connections, such as between type of beaks and types of food available. With no detail of context the explanation that a change is adaptive is bordering on the preformationist, 'If it exists, it must have been adaptive', being given as the explanation of the adaptation, with no independent evidence of adaptive value. Even a view like that of Gabora and Colgan, in which it is claimed that adaptations are relatively specific solutions to specific problems, like avoiding predators or obtaining energy, is wide open to criticism because although 'avoiding predators' is an understandable logical category, it is a meaningless ecological category because it is an abstraction. It is not grounded in the material world of specific events as it specifies no particular predator in no particular contexts and therefore no real material situation in which success or otherwise could be an outcome. Ideas cannot be selected, only material states and events in particular contexts.

Consider a prey trying to escape by running down a burrow. A successful outcome depends upon it being able to perceive when the predator is nearby, where the burrow is, being able to navigate quickly and accurately towards the burrow, not to mention being small enough to fit, having means of locomotion, etc. But it also depends upon the characteristics of the prey, the fact that it cannot go down burrows, that it can perceive you and catch you, etc. Both sorts of capacities are a mixture of phylogenetic and ontogenetic considerations, as the evolved visual powers of the predator, for instance, are brought to bear, while the particular experiences of this escaper aid or inhibit survival. But even the skills, attributes, limitations of each are only part of the story because what is critical here is the relation between the powers of the prey and of the predator, for a given physical situation. Suppose our predator is a fast digger, or comes to be able to get down burrows, the whole 'game' may change. Just as the reliable co-occurrence of genes and external contexts has been identified as crucial for development, so we can now begin to see that what is selected in this scenario has to be the reliable co-occurrence of all the relations between predator and prey. Change one aspect, the rest may have to reorganize. The means of avoiding predators is thus determined by the powers or affordances the predator has, those the prey has, and these include those arising from the relations of the prey and the predator to the physical geography. The physics of the body of the prey and of the predator and the geography combine together to determine whether a given sort of behaviour will be adaptive. The unit of selection is all of these.

Look what happens if it is not, if one factor is changed. We could have an animal that was brilliant at disappearing down burrows, but not when the predator appeared, or brilliant at running when it appeared, but not down burrows, or brilliant at perceiving predator and burrow, but failing to run. None of these are of any use, none can be adaptive, and thus selected, because the only thing that can be adaptive is the *systematic combination* of the perception of the predator, the perception of location of burrow, and the act of getting down it quickly, given the predator dynamics.

A different species has different characteristics and so even if preyed on by the same bird of prey may need to make use of different affordances, e.g. camouflage, because the pattern of relations is different. If burrows disappeared it is surely clear that the whole system by which predator avoidance (and thus prey capture by the bird as well) for this species of prey and predator could completely change. It would become reorganised to 'take account' of all the sorts of factors we have been talking about. The developmental system itself evolved in the face of this dynamic complexity.

The Retention of Preformationist Thinking

I want now to offer some thoughts about the ways in which their thinking appears to be constrained by the traditional assumptions, and to offer an alternative. First, the location of information. This is what Johnson and Morton have to say about the primal mechanism. It is:

A cognitive mechanism *in the neonate's brain* [emphasis mine] with the following properties:

- The mechanism contains structural information concerning the visual characteristics possessed by conspecifics. By 'structural' we mean that the information is concerned with relative spatial position of elements within a pattern. We use the term Conspec for the device, since it specifies conspecifics in the context of the species-typical environment.
- As the relevant biological event that occurs is the movement of the infant face to see and follow the species-typical face, and it occurs after an interaction, between the external species-typical input and some part of the (species-typical) brain, we should conclude that information arises from the interaction, and is not usefully said to be preformed in the brain, or anywhere else. Johnson and Morton are de-emphasizing the need for coupled internal and external structure to co-exist and interact for relevant outcomes to occur and emphasizing a preformation of information. They are writing as if there is a preformed internal structure against which external structure is compared (how?) till a match is made and as if one component of an interaction could produce information on its own.

Lack of Appreciation of the Equal Status of Interacting Factors

Johnson and Morton refer on many occasions to the 'speciestypical environment'. They always mean the external environment. But the internal species-typical environment, part of the brain in this instance, is equally important. The adaptive movement of the head is the outcome of the interaction of aspects of the external and internal species typical contexts. The focus on just one component in this interaction inhibits the appreciation that it is in and only in the interaction between organism and environment that adaptive outcomes emerge and that both sorts of components have equal status in this interaction.

The Coupling of Perception and Action and the Issue of Representation

There is also an undue emphasis upon the purely perceptual aspects of the process. The description of Conspec refers only to the visual characteristics of a human face. But without the infant tracking the moving image, no adaptive change can accrue. For an adaptive outcome, movement was required and movement was duly produced. As I have tried to emphasize, a perceptual ability on its own could not be selected, as it is only action-in-context which works or doesn't. Johnson and Morton may be led to describe what goes on in terms of the neonate having a built-in knowledge of the human face because they accept the basic assumption that representations are the key to action. And they may be committed to that view because they conceive of perception and cognition and action as separate first there is an act of perception, then the brain makes a decision about what is really out there, cognition, then it makes a decision about what to do about it, action. This is still standard thinking, consistent with a view of psychological processes as independent of each other, not coupled as an ecological view would assume. In my view we cannot infer that there is a representation of a face in the brain. And we don't need to. What we can infer is that some structure, some invariances are 'picked up' by the neonate and that these are directly coupled to action in respect of that input. There is no need to speculate about the nature of inner processes, what matters is to state the relation between what is in the environment and what the infant does about it. What has been selected is the turning of head to a specific contextual item when that item is encountered. It is initially no different to a gull chick's peck. It becomes different, because, as we shall see later, humans can de-couple action and thought.

The Failure to Explore the Dyad as the Unit of Analysis

Johnson and Morton also pay little attention to the actions of the mother in this scenario, focusing completely on a structure in the head of the neonate. But the 'preference' for the species-typical face may be just as much due to actions by the mother to manipulate the attention systems of the newborn, her positioning and actions affording highly interesting and information-rich input, as Bushnell suggests. Certainly her actions are important, though the fact that the neonates did track a two-dimensional model of a face on a 'bat' moving, hardly the ultimate in salient input, suggests that is also not the whole story. Rather, if the dyadic system is the unit of analysis, it follows that we see the actions of both parties as equally important. Remember, we cannot reasonably infer that the main causal power resides in the organism or the environment. In this case the main element of the environment is an organism, usually mother, but the logic is the same, causal outcomes only emerge from the flux of interactions involving organism and environment, and the system of dyadic interaction is the unit of selection here, not the acts of a component.

Change as Continuous, not Dichotomous

Johnson and Morton also appear to retain a dichotomous view of the sorts of changes that occur in the process of development : either the change is species-typical and unlearned, or it is individual-specific and learned. There is no recognition that the process may involve a gradually increasing differentiation of the environment. But consider this evidence. Walton, Bower and Bower, for instance, obtained higher amplitude sucking to produce a video of mother's face at 12-36 hours, compared with a face that was not mother's, and Bushnell reports several other studies showing recognition of something that functioned to discriminate between mother and another. But these results are explained by realizing that it is probably only differences in shape of head and hair that are the basis for differentiation in the first days. At two months physiognomic differences are the basis of preference. That is, it is important to see development as a gradual increase in differentiation, as changes along a continuum, rather than in terms of an unlearned/learned dichotomy.

The 'Generic/specific' Continuum of Knowledge

Johnson and Morton seem to focus on the unlearned speciestypical aspect of the first primal interaction, as if its relation to 'innateness' was important. Given what I have suggested about the importance of generic constraints or effects on subsystems, I suggest the orientation should be mainly regarded as involving relatively undifferentiated perceptual, cognitive and motor abilities which result in limiting learning, focusing in certain areas, without specifically determining exactly what is learned. The learning that does occur will involve a variety of more specific, differentiated information, for example about particular aspects of communication, about self and others in interaction, about intermodality. These are more differentiated sorts of knowledge than is involved in the generic preference for faces, but all afforded by, made possible by, the constraining effect of the narrowing of attention, the limiting of what is perceived and thus available for learning about. This is our first concrete example in human development of the principle that generic interactions produce knowledge at a relatively undifferentiated level, such knowledge enabling new interactions at lower levels which provide more differentiated and specific knowledge.

The Multiple Affordances of Primal Interactions

Johnson and Morton focus on only one function of the primal act, to aid recognition learning. But systems are messy. Attention to the face of a significant caregiver affords the best opportunities for the infant and the caregiver to gain maximal information about the state of the person they are with; it affords viewing of the movements of the face, the eyes, the mouth, movements in space and time; it does so for the caregiver as well and as this means the two can perceive their own and the others acts, it means learning about contingencies in interaction can occur, the perception of 'turn-taking', for instance, being afforded; it also affords the chance to notice contingencies between the different behaviours of the 'other', such as the changing shape of their mouth as they speak, the changing of their expression as their voice changes (in tension, in relaxation), etc. This single example of a primal interaction shows how a simple movement, orientation to a face, can afford significant and complex development opportunities. It also points to the dangers of the interaction not taking place, though it may be that there are other means of obtaining the preferential attention.

Different Extensions of Invariance within the Same 'Stimulus'

There is a developmental aspect to this research which is again not focused on by Johnson and Morton. They refer to the species-typical input of a human face, but the fact is that what is perceived itself follows a developmental pathway.

It shows how the same face might appear to a newborn compared to how it appears to someone with high visual acuity, which is the same as saying how it will normally appear to the same person later in their development. The external invariances constituting the species-typical face are less differentiated than those required for personal identification in the individual-specific interactions. At one point in development the former invariances are informative while the latter are not, but the operation of the former enables interactions by which the latter become informative. The process of development itself transforms the external environment. It becomes what it was not. Again, there are not two faces, but a continuum of them, the differentiation gradually emerging. The 'same' face is many faces.

Moreover, further thought again demonstrates the integration of what is 'species-typical' (related to nature) and what is specific (related to nurture), as follows. A species-typical face has invariances which are not specific to an individual, so what to look at can be known by the undifferentiated interaction, but where to look can be known only by a differentiated interaction, because the face is in an exact position. Part of the mechanism must thus be sensitive to this aspect of local context, position and movement, and part to the species-typical context. For successful completion of the first part of the task, the infant must not only utilize the invariances specifying that there is a species-typical human about, that is, the 'what' problem must be sorted, it must also specify where it is in order to attend to it, thus solving the 'where' problem. The 'what' is dependent upon utilization of extensions which have lasted over speciestypical space and time, the 'where' by extensions of seconds and centimetres. This is another example of phylogenetic and ontogenetic factors being integrated, of 'nature' and 'nurture', interacting in systematic ways to utilize the invariances in the environment. Species-typical actions have to include this 'sensitive-to-this-moment' aspect for them to work.

Variations in Faces and the Interacting Factors Involved

As the differences between faces constitutes a nice example of how there is no dichotomy between faces as 'species-typical' or 'unique'. It is not only the phenomenal face that varies with development, actual faces also vary to some extent according to racial origin, an extension of invariance between species-typical and individual. But then we will think of family resemblances, another extension of invariance. But faces also vary according to age, an interesting case in that there is a species-typical aspect to the change for the species during life (the change is relatively invariant for the species), and an individual aspect. You may well now be thinking that there are gender differences as well, and then move on to conjecture how species, racial, age, gender, familial, aspects of facial invariance interact with each other and with external environmental contingencies. Thus, there are great variations between instances of what is still invariant enough for it to be recognised by all, a face, and variations in the extent to which we can extract invariances coupled to ones developmental level, not mention quality of vision, etc. This is what dynamic theories appreciate, the nature of complexity, the amazing amount of variation, of interaction and yet of stability as well. The emphasis on a simple learned/not learned dichotomy signally fails to do justice to what we actually encounter.

The Effects of Non-obvious Early Experience

Johnson and Morton seem to suggest that nothing relevant to preferences or to other primal interactions occurs before birth. This itself may be linked to the traditional idea that the neonate is incompetent and that nothing useful for cognitive development could have previously occurred. Far from it. Prenatal experience is particularly relevant in so far as it involves the first searches of task spaces, the first attempts to act in and on their world which, of course, the developing infant does not know is going to change dramatically at about nine months. All such motor and perceptual (especially but not only auditory) experience, and thereby reorganisation, learning, are precursors to and conditions of, later differentiation. Given also that we shall find strong evidence that information in one mode is informative for other modes, so that, for instance, movement of one's own face in the womb can be 'recognized' when the infant sees another face, the conclusion has to be that a great deal of relevant experience has already occurred before birth and that again the notion of a continuum of differentiation is more relevant than the dichotomy between what is learned and what is not.

Gottlieb and others have found evidence in birds which demonstrates the significance of prenatal, perceptual experience. One case involves wood ducklings. He found they failed to show a preference for their mother's call after hatching unless they had heard, whilst still in the egg, the alarm call of their siblings, and that it was a specific aspect of that call that was critical, a drop in frequency towards the end of the call, which was very similar to the adult mother's call. With mallard ducklings it was their own call they needed to hear, but in both cases he found that the function, the effect of the initial auditory experience, was to reduce the range of frequency of input to which the duckling was sensitive. Because 'mother's' call was within this range, whilst other ducks calls were not, this effectively meant that they normally heard their mothers call, but not that of other species and thus did react to mother and did not react to the calls of other species.

Sleigh, Columbus and Lickliter found that bobtail quail chicks which were exposed to species-typical, maternal auditory input (mother's call) but not simultaneously to species-typical maternal visual input (sight of mother) did not develop a preference for the sight and sound of 'mother' over the sight of a different species of quail hen emitting the bobwhite call. The experience of concurrent maternal auditory and visual input was necessary for the later preference to be shown. These cases show that 'primal' interactions may depend not only on upon relevant environmental input at the time, but on earlier, even more undifferentiated (even more primal) interactions. So even interactions which we are only just coming to accept as requiring relevant input, not being 'innate', may depend upon previous, non-obvious experience.

Two: Disembedded Mind or Embedded Robot

The serial computer metaphor: why it is so powerful, but why it is so wrong.

In this first case I want to show how the general metaphor of the human mind as akin to a serial computer served, serves still, to help maintain preformationist and dichotomous thinking, by itself being based upon the same assumptions. We begin with the uncontroversial notion of the human as a brilliant information processor, like a computer but much, much better. Humans process raw perceptual data, use a central set of representations to classify it and make decisions, and carry out the appropriate behaviour. So do serial computers. They input data into the appropriate format, find solutions through the application of the central programme, and decode the decision into the designated form of output or print-out. In addition, both the serial computer and the mature human mind operate with symbols, an abstract formal code, with the resultant power to classify and categorize in terms of criterial qualities and to operate in a 'disembedded' manner, not being tied to specific contexts or instances. Moreover, just as serial computers carry out separate, successive information-processing operations and sends the processed data, as so often indicated on a flow chart, to the next processing unit, so humans have the separate processes of perception, cognition and action by which intelligent action is achieved. For some years it was accepted by all but a tiny minority of stalwarts that this was a most useful way to conceive of the functioning of the human mind, that its structure and functioning was basically of the same general sort as a serial computer.

A key feature here is the relation of perception, cognition and action to each other. In human development the assumption is that individual acts of perception can only reveal appearances, while acts of cognition, using concepts (symbols and the like) reveal reality. Perception is thus totally separate from cognition, merely providing raw, basic data for the complex representational structures to analyze and make sense of. The ability to use concepts thus allows one to be sure that any particular instance of, for instance, a sexist act, or a hedgehog, can be correctly classified and not mistaken because a decision was based only upon its appearance which will include contextual, 'interfering' features. Input to computers similarly has no role in complex thinking, it merely gives the programme something to work with, raw data. There is an absolutely clear distinction between raw data and the programme, the software, just as there is between perception and cognition in the traditional model. Similarly, the output from a computer is disconnected from the complex analysis of data, being merely a form of presentation of results, a digital print-out, graphs, statistical tables, the written word, whatever. Computer output has to be the analogue of behaviour, so again the metaphor is taken to be apt because action and output are not where complexity lie, because that is back in the programme. The same sort of thinking extends to buildings, etc. We understand that when we are told that a certain bridge or palace was built by a famous individual, we know that what we are intended to understand is that the complicated, intelligent work, the design, was done by this person, and the names of those who did build it is irrelevant. The output is connected to the processing in one direction only, it is directed by it but has no direct effect on it. The 'hub', all the complexity, is based in the central programme. Both perception and action, input and output, have the same epistemological status and function in the production of knowledge very low.

But humans and indeed many species show amazing skill in adapting sensitively to variation in the physical or mental terrain, subtle abilities to cope with unexpected environmental contingencies throughout their lives. Indeed, intelligent action is precisely that which does show the ability to sensitively adjust to new situations and which is not stereotyped and rigid in its form. This sensitivity to context, this coupling of organism and environment in action, is emphasized in the ecological view. Each organism must be able to perceive the salient features of its environment, must know what context it is operating in in order to act according to particular conditions. And as situations change, the ability to notice this and react to it must be part of the design. Now how can this be ensured? The simple and compelling answer is that there must be a strong and permanent coupling maintained between its action systems, its perceptual systems and its cognitive systems. Only in this way can the organism maintain sensitivity to change and do something about it. When this is the way functioning is organized we are seeing a system in action, the organism-inenvironment system. It is systems which need to be understood and the individual organism is part of an ecosystem. This much is accepted, part of espoused theory and yet we retain a metaphor for thinking based upon the exact opposite.

The conclusion has to be that the concept of ecology simply has no relevance to this information processor. It is the only intelligent thing that ever existed that did not have to display a sensitive relation to its ecology and in which the cleverness was nothing to do with its actual effect on the material environment, but only on what was inside. It is a powerful but lonely organism. It is a mind conceived as superior to its environment, imposing order on it and orders about it through its physical outputs.

The metaphor was and is widely accepted because it reinforces the underlying assumption that the character of the internal, preformed, complex mental processes is basically unrelated to the particular contexts from which they derive, namely, material action in the material world.

The computer software is the mind, the hardware is the body. In the mature mind, what the body does does not affect the complexity of the mind. In the complex programme the output does not affect the programme. The software makes sense of raw data. Cognition makes sense of perceptual data. The mind imposes meaning on an otherwise meaningless world. It is boss. The body merely carries out what it is ordered to do. In short, the metaphor reinforces the 'mind/body' dichotomy. It does the same for 'nature/nurture'. 'Nature' corresponds to the simple, bodily hardware functions, 'nurture' to the complex mental ones, distinct from the hardware. Hence we find that the supposedly archaic notion of preformation never left the serial computer the programme is the homunculus, the 'mind' of the computer, rendering bodily action (print-out) and perception (raw material data) redundant in the production of knowledge.

None of this implies that the design of computers has to be totally different to people. Now going to describe a computer in which perception, cognition and action are closely coupled. It is one without a complex central programme. In fact its starting points are positively feeble. In so far as it has a programme at all, it simply links its sensing (perception) to its outputs (action) and records what it does. It is a parallel processor, not a serial processor, based upon a connectionist mode of thinking. And yet its performance turns out to be pretty impressive, absolutely impossible according to the traditional view. It proves that complexity can emerge without complex built-in representations, that preformation is not necessary, that mind and body, nature and nurture, can be united.

Connectionism

I add here a note about connectionist modelling, because I think it is hard to grasp. It is based upon totally different assumptions to that of serial processing in that the computer is not given a predetermined (preformed) programme. Instead, it is limited to a few basic rules which can be varied by the experimenter to see what difference different starting points make to the emergence of the state of the model. The model consists of electrical systems with nodes, points at which inputs arrive and outputs leave. There are various sorts of nodes in a model. When exposed to input, activity results and currents flow in various directions, through various nodes. It is then repeatedly exposed to patterns of input, and variations to the 'rules' like which nodes connect to which others or with what likelihood, are made to maximize the similarity of the computer output with the input to it. What is amazing is that complex programmes emerge, exactly as if the programme had been given complex representations to start with. In addition, the development of the programme often 'mimics' the abrupt developmental transitions observed in humans. The only way this can happen is if there was complexity in the structure of the environment in the first place, because apart from some not complex rules, that is the only source of information the model has. All the complex structures, like grammatical rules, which have been found to emerge in connectionist models can be accounted for only by acknowledging that these external structures (what we shall later call 'higher-order invariances') can be picked up by models which are sensitive to input. It is like the robot. Its ability to get about and have a map and select routes were based upon its ability to detect input, from its sensors and its own movement. That is all that is required. You will find that this ability to detect external structure, to 'pick up' invariance, is exactly what the foremost ecological psychologist, J.J. Gibson, wrote that people could do. Thus, ecological and systems thinking is not anti-computational, but it is anticompartmental, anti-dichotomies.

We become acquainted with the key features of one of the two existing areas of theorizing and empirical research which should illuminate the ecological, systems thinking about development, dynamic systems views.

7

Cognitive Development

Introduction

One thing a reader new to the field is likely to gain from this chapter is an appreciation of why the study of cognitive development has not yielded simple, straightforward answers to seemingly simple, straightforward, empirically researchable questions. For example, does basic memory capacity increase or remain constant as the individual develops? The reader should come to appreciate why such questions themselves, as well as their answers, turn out to be considerably more complex than they appear on the surface. Although the reader new to the field may be disillusioned to learn that the field lacks simple, easily answered research questions or an accumulated body of perspective-free facts, I argue in this chapter that there is actually considerable reason to be optimistic regarding the field's past and prospective progress. As suggested later on, the field is in many ways at a turning point in its own development, with considerable promise for future progress. A number of long-standing polarities, controversies, and preoccupations that have detracted attention from the central questions crucial to an understanding of cognitive development have in recent years either been resolved, set aside, or recast, with the result that attention is now focused more directly on these key questions. Some might take the negative view that through the succession of windows in terms of which it has proceeded, the field has done no more that repeat itself and, in effect, stand still. I take exception to this view and suggest instead ways in which these windows are becoming clearer as the perspectives they entail increase in explanatory power.

Coordination of Mind and Reality: Basic Perspectives

An adequate account of cognitive development must, at a minimum, contain answers to two basic questions: What is it that develops? How does this development occur? The answer to the first question, at least, might appear obvious: The profound differences in the intellectual functions exhibited by the newborn infant and the mature adult are evident to the most casual observer. It is this development that is the obvious object of concern. In fact, the different theoretical and methodological approaches to the study of cognitive development that I examine represent a wide variety of views as to what is developing, ranging from individual stimulus response connections to discrete, context-linked skills, to a smaller set of more general cognitive functions, to a single broad system of cognitive operations that underlies all more specific intellectual abilities and behaviours.

The second question also harbors greater complexity than is suggested on the surface. There is more to be explained than how intellectual functioning, or mind, is transformed during the course of development, though formulating such an explanation is in itself a formidable challenge. The full question that must be addressed, rather, is how the mind develops *in the particular direction*, or toward the particular end, that it does, rather than in a host of other possible directions, so as to become well-adapted to the external world of which the developing individual is a part. The two questions are, of course, not independent. The answer to the second question to a large degree determines the answer to the first, though the reverse is less true. In the following discussion, therefore, I focus on answers to the second question, noting their implications with respect to the first question.

Three broad answers to the second question have appeared and reappeared throughout the history of developmental psychology. All three, in fact, have their roots in classical philosophical traditions that predate psychology as a field of scientific study. Each of the perspectives can be classified in terms of which of these three answers it reflects.

The first answer, rooted in the philosophical tradition known as rationalism, is that mind and reality exist in pre-established coordination with one another. In other words, the particular direction in which the mind will develop is predetermined, presumably through some form of genetic coding unique to the species. The second answer, whose roots lie in the philosophical tradition known as empiricism, is that the nature of reality is imposed on the mind from without during the course of development, and it is for this reason that mind and reality come to coordinate with one another. The third answer, rooted in the philosophical tradition known as interactionism, is that mind is neither in pre-established coordination with reality nor molded by it from without; rather, through a lengthy series of interchanges between individual and environment, the coordination is gradually achieved.

Maturationism

The first of the three answers is reflected in the first theoretical perspective to have a major guiding influence on the study of child development by North American psychologists, the doctrine of maturationism. Until the appearance of the work by Arnold Gesell, the major advocate of maturationism, studies of children's development had been conducted largely within the atheoretical "child study movement" that flourished in America during the early part of the twentieth century. It can be argued that the myriad of descriptive studies of children's knowledge and interests produced by the child study movement did not make a lasting contribution to our understanding precisely because these investigations were not guided by an overarching conceptual framework. Gesell's studies, in strong contrast, adhere clearly to a mold dictated by his theoretical view.

Gesell was struck by the regularity he observed in the emergence of various motor abilities during the first years of life, despite huge variability in environmental circumstances. These observations led him to posit that new skills emerge according to a regular sequence and timetable that are the product of a predetermined genetic code, similar, for example, to the code that governs the appearance of secondary sexual characteristics at puberty. Maturation, Gesell proposed, is the internal regulatory mechanism that governs the emergence of all new skills and abilities cognitive as well as behavioural that appear with advancing age. Thus, according to this view, it is a sequence of discrete skills that develops, and the mechanism by means of which this development occurs is one of predetermined unfolding.

Gesell and his coworkers engaged in meticulous cross-sectional and longitudinal observations of infants, which enabled them to describe in precise detail the sequence and timetable in terms of which early motor abilities appeared. Subsequent bodies of such research in developmental psychology have been criticized as "merely descriptive," but one cannot lodge this criticism against Gesell's work, for there is a logical link between his research strategy and his theory: If the appearance of new behaviours is the product of an innate genetic code, the researcher's task is merely to provide a precise description of this unfolding; no further explanation is necessary.

An experimental methodology would seem to have no place in Gesell's work. One experiment Gesell performed, however, has become a classic. Gesell conducted the experiment for the purpose of demonstrating the secondary role of the environment, relative to the central role he believed is played by the process of maturation. Quite unlike most modem experiments, Gesell's experiment had only two subjects, 11-month-old twin girls. At the onset of the experiment, neither twin exhibited any proficiency in the skill that was to be the focus of the experiment: stair climbing. Gesell proceeded to subject one of the twins to daily training sessions on a specially constructed staircase for a period of six weeks. At the end of this period, the trained twin was a proficient stair climber, while the control (untrained) twin still showed no ability.

At this point, the experiment would appear to show exactly the opposite of what Gesell held; i.e., it appears to show that the acquisition of motor skills is highly susceptible to environmental influence. The experiment did not end at this point, however. Several weeks later, the control twin spontaneously began to exhibit some stair climbing proficiency. At this point, Gesell instituted a two week period of training of the same type that had been administered to the experimental twin. At the end of this period, the control twin equaled her experimental twin in stair climbing proficiency, and the two remained equivalent in proficiency from then on.

What Gesell wished to demonstrate by this experiment, of course, is that the environment, or "experience," plays at most a superficial, secondary role in temporarily accelerating the emergence of a skill that is destined by the maturational code to appear at a later time. While these results were initially accepted by some as evidence of the correctness of Gesell's maturational doctrine, a major criticism of the experiment was raised. Did the experimental design adequately control for the effects of experience? The untrained twin continued to have experience of a variety of sorts, even if it was not stair climbing, during the period the experimental twin was being trained. Could this experience legitimately be ruled out as having contributed to the eventual appearance of the untrained twin's skill?

At first, the issue was regarded as a problem in research design. Were it feasible on both ethical and technical grounds to totally restrict the experience of the control twin during the training period, then experience could be ruled out as a contributing factor. Ultimately, however, the problem was recognized as a logical, not a methodological, one. As long as an organism has life, it is always undergoing some experience, by the very definition of what it is to be alive. Thus, a process of maturation can be observed only in the case of a living organism that is undergoing experience of some sort during the period of observation. It is, in turn, impossible to rule out this experience as having played a role in the emergence of new behaviours exhibited by the organism.

Following this recognition of the impossibility of eliminating experience as a contributing factor to development, interest in the maturational doctrine declined, and attention turned instead toward investigating how this experience influences development. Few, if any, current developmental psychologists would categorize themselves as maturationists. The modern-day theorist to whom the maturationist (or, to use the more common modern term, nativist) view is most often attributed is the linguist Chomsky. It is important to note, however, that Chomsky does not subscribe to a nativist doctrine in anything like the strong sense of Gesell. Chomsky regards the *capacity* to acquire language as an innate capacity that is unique to the human organism (in contrast to Piaget, who regards the capacity for language as evolving out of sensorimotor activity during infancy). Chomsky (as well as Piaget), however, regards experience as an essential aspect of the *process* of language acquisition.

The pure doctrine of maturationism, then, is significant because of its historical influence, rather than as a guiding perspective in the current study of cognitive development. Rejection of the doctrine of maturationism, it should be emphasized, however, does not imply the rejection of underlying physical or neurological changes as critical to the emergence of new cognitive or behavioural skills. On the contrary, developments in the brain and nervous system that appear to be critical for behavioural development have become a topic of intense interest and research effort in recent years. These physical developments, however, do not by themselves initiate related behavioural developments. At most, they are enabling conditions that make it possible for the behavioural developments to take place; the process of behavioural development itself remains to be explained.

Empiricism

Although Gesell's studies were theoretically motivated, his descriptions of developmental patterns were attended to more for their practical than their theoretical significance, as the field at this point, under the influence of the child study movement, was still very practically oriented. In fact, the series of books by Gesell and his co-workers that describe developmental norms for parents and teachers are still referred to today. It is probably accurate to say, then, that when the empiricist movement that had come to occupy the mainstream of academic psychology by the middle of this century embraced the field of child development, it was the first time that the field's research efforts became dominated by an overarching theoretical framework.

The empiricist view represented a striking counterinfluence following Gesell's maturationism. If developmental change does not arise from within the organism, then perhaps it is imposed from without by the environment. This solution represents the second of the three answers referred to earlier: Mind and reality come to be coordinated with one another because reality imposes itself on, and hence shapes, the mind over the course of development. Mind, then, is in the beginning Locke's classic *tabula rasa*, or blank slate.

The name of B.F. Skinner is the one most closely identified with the empiricist doctrine known as behaviourism that dominated the study of psychology in North America for several decades. Skinner explored the full implications of the Law of Effect originally proposed by Thorndike at the turn of the century: Organisms tend to repeat those behaviours that have satisfying consequences and to eliminate those that do not. Thus, the behaviours an organism comes to exhibit are a direct function of their environmental consequences. The organism is thereby shaped by its environment.

Bijou and Baer are the two theorists most widely known for applying Skinner's doctrine to the realm of child development. The child, they have proposed, is most appropriately conceptualized as "a cluster of interrelated responses". Development, in turn, consists of the progressive shaping of these individual responses by the environment. Like Skinner, Bijou and Baer held as one of their most important tenets that the temptation of relying on unobservable internal constructs to explain behaviour must be avoided. Only external, observable behaviours are the proper object of scientific study. The observable behaviours, in turn, are a function of observable external events. To speculate about processes internal to the individual only obscures the direct connection between external behaviour and the external stimuli that control it.

One might wonder what relevance such a doctrine could have for the study of cognition and its development, as cognition almost by definition is a process that occurs within the individual. Bijou and Baer, however, took the position that cognition is nothing more than a particular class of behaviour and, as such, it is under the same environmental control as any other behaviour. For example, consider what (mistakenly) might be regarded as an internal concept that a young child has of, say, animal. What this so-called "concept" actually consists of, according to Bijou and Baer, is a common behavioural response the child has learned to exhibit (as a function of external reinforcement) in the presence of objects or events that have a certain set of properties (e.g., movement, four legs, eyes, nose, mouth, perhaps fur or tail). It is thus not fruitful to regard the concept as either inside the child's head or existing in nature. Rather, such "conceptual" behaviour is under the control of the environmental agents that administer the apprcpriate reinforcement contingencies (i.e., signify approval if the child emits the response when the defining properties are present). It could well be a different set of properties (and hence a different "conceptual" behaviour) that the agents chose to reinforce.

A few fundamental principles have governed research in cognitive development that is carried out within the empiricist framework. The most important are the principle of reductionism, the related principle of parsimony, and the principle of experimental control. Reductionism has been influential both as a theoretical principle and as a research strategy. As a theoretical principle, reductionism is the assertion that any complex behaviour is in fact a constellation of very simple behaviours. As a research strategy, reductionism dictates that the smallest possible behavioural units that make up a complex behaviour be isolated and investigated individually. Once the process governing each of these individual units is understood, explanations of more complex forms of behaviour should follow.

The related principles of parsimony holds that an explanatory mechanism that accounts for the broadest range of phenomena is to be preferred over one that accounts for a narrower range of phenomena. In the case of behaviourist theory, this has meant that more complex explanations must be rejected if a behaviour can be accounted for in terms of the simple mechanism of operant conditioning; that is, control by means of external reinforcement. Applied to the field of developmental psychology, the major implication of the principle of parsimony is that developmental phenomena can (and should) be regarded as the accumulated effects of the operation of the simple conditioning (or learning) mechanism. In other words, development can be reduced to the simpler process of learning. Hence, there is no need to retain the more complex term.

The parsimony principle is also reflected in the assumption that the basic learning mechanism functions in an identical way throughout an individual's development. One implication of this assumption with respect to research strategy is that there is no need to compare individuals at different points in their development. If a particular learning process is observed to operate at one age level, it is assumed that it will operate in the same way at any other age level. Thus, researchers studying cognitive development within an empiricist framework have tended to utilize a single age group in their studies. Rarely have they engaged in the cross-sectional and longitudinal age comparisons that characterize much developmental research.

The principle of experimental control has led to the almost exclusive choice of an experimental laboratory method. As the laboratory provides a controlled environment, the researcher can introduce the environmental variable believed to control a particular behaviour in order to establish that it does in fact produce that behaviour, with reasonable assurance that it is not some other (uncontrolled) variable that has actually produced the behaviour, which might be the case in a natural setting.

A research programme conducted within the empiricist framework that illustrates all of these principles is the laboratory study of paired-associate learning that was prevalent in the 1950s and 1960s. In a paired-associate learning experiment, a subject is exposed to pairs of nonsense syllables (e.g., PIF and LER) until a connection is established between the two members of the pair, such that the presentation of one syllable enables the subject to recite the other. The choice of arbitrary (nonsensical) material to be learned is not itself arbitrary but rather is an important part of the research strategy, dictated by the objective of experimental control. Arbitrary associations between meaningless syllables will be completely, and therefore equally, new to all learners. Individual differences in past learning and reinforcement are controlled for in this manner.

Paired-associate learning experiments were conducted both with children of different ages and with adults as subjects. The purpose of these experiments, however, was not to compare the performance of different age groups. Rather, the large number of studies conducted were all devoted to identifying the variables (for example, exposure time or distinctiveness of syllables) that affect the learning process; it was assumed that these variables would function in an identical way for all subjects.

The tremendous effort devoted to the study of paired-associate learning was justified on the assumption that it represents one of the simplest, most basic forms of learning, and that understanding how it operates would provide a key to understanding the more complex and significant forms of learning that occur in schools and other natural settings. To critics who argue that it would be preferable to devote research efforts to studying these more complex forms of learning directly, proponents of the reductionist strategy counter that the learning that occurs in natural contexts is simply too complex to be amenable to investigation. Employing the reductionist strategy, they would claim, provides the only avenue to eventual understanding.

The maturationist and empiricist perspectives that have been described in this chapter reflect two of the three answers to the basic question posed at the outset: How does the mind develop so as to become coordinated with the external world it inhabits? The answers that underlie these two perspectives are diametrically opposed. The maturationist answer is that this coordination is pre-established within the individual, and the empiricist answer is that this coordination is imposed on the individual by the external world. Let us turn now to the perspective that reflects the third of these answers.

Piaget and Constructivism

American developmental psychology was in many ways ripe for its "discovery" of Piaget in the 1950s. The Piagetian influence brought something new that many would argue had been conspicuously absent in the study of the child's cognitive (as well as social) development: the "rediscovery of the child's mind," as one observer (Martin, 1959/60) put it at the time. Some would g so far as to claim that the study of cognitive development began with Piaget; before Piaget, there existed a psychology of learning, not a psychology of development. Many of Piaget's ideas are evident in the work of the philosopher and psychologist, James Mark Baldwin, as well as Piaget's contemporary, Heinz Werner. Yet it was Piaget who was to have the major influence on the study of cognitive development in psychology, even though his scholarly career had been under way in Europe for several decades before American psychologists became interested in his work.

Piaget's descriptions of "childish" thought intrigued a wide audience of psychologists and educators. Young children's beliefs that the amount of liquid changes when poured into a differently-shaped container; that names are a part of the objects they represent; that the sun follows one around and thinks and feels as humans do; that one's own thoughts and dreams are material objects visible to observers; to cite a few of the most well-known examples, were startling revelations to many who regarded themselves as knowledgeable about children. These features of children's thought evidently had been "there to be seen" for centuries, but in most cases had never been noted before.

Piaget, however, found these observations of childish thought significant not so much for their own sake as for their implications regarding the mechanisms by which the mind develops. If asked to draw the liquid as it would appear while the container is tilted at a 45-degree angle, young children tend not to represent the liquid by a line parallel to the true horizontal. Instead, they draw the line showing the liquid parallel to the top and bottom of the container. No child has ever seen liquid in a container in that way. The child's drawing, therefore, cannot be a direct reflection of his or her experience with objects and events in the physical world. Instead, Piaget argued, it must be an intellectual construction the child's understanding of what he or she sees.

Each observation of this sort was significant in Piaget's view as testimony to the fact that the child is engaged in an extended intellectual "meaning making" endeavor. In other words, the child is attempting to construct an understanding of self, other, and the world of objects. "Childish" beliefs, such as nonconservation (e.g., of the true horizontal, following a perceptual alteration such as the tilting of the container, or of quantity, following transfer to a differently-shaped container), are significant because they cannot have been directly internalized from the external world. Nor is it plausible that these beliefs are innate and simply appear, uninfluenced by the child's experience in the world.

In discounting these opposing alternatives, Piaget proposed at least the general form of a third solution to the question of how mind and reality come to be coordinated with one another. Through a process of organism-environment, or subject-object, interchanges, the subject gradually constructs an understanding of both its own actions and the external world. The most important feature of this interchange is that it is bidirectional: The organism and the external world gradually come to "fit" one another neither makes any radical or unilateral accommodations to the other. Each new "childish belief" that is discovered, i.e., each new belief that directly reflects neither the external world nor the child's innate disposition, provides further evidence of the occurrence of this bidirectional interchange and, hence, constructive process.

Doctrine of Stages

It has been suggested that the single, most central idea in Piaget's wide ranging theory is that the intellectual effort to understand one's own actions and their relation to the world of objects i.e.. the individual's extended "meaning making" enterprise motivates, or energizes, a constructive process directed toward progressively greater equilibrium between the individual and the environment. Thus, when Piaget's influence became prominent in American psychology, one might have expected that it would be this constructive, meaning making enterprise, or at the very least the "rediscovery of the child's mind," that Piaget would represent.

Instead, it was the derivative doctrine of stages that came to identify Piaget's theory in developmental psychology. The individual's meaning-making effort, Piaget believed, was marked by a striving for coherence, with the result that the individual's ideas had a unity to them, even if the ideas were largely incorrect by external, or mature, standards. In other words, these ideas were reflections of a broad, unified cognitive system that had its own unique form and that mediated all of the more specific manifestations of the individual's cognitive functioning.

Furthermore, it was this cognitive system as a whole that allegedly underwent developmental change. As a result of the interactive process directed toward adaptation, or greater equilibrium between organism and environment, the cognitive system underwent a series of major reorganisations, each reflecting an improved equilibrium mind and reality were better coordinated than they had been previously. These newly and better organized mental structures, or "stages," were held to appear in an invariant sequence universal to the human species. Each new structure reflected the most probable organisation to emerge from the organism environment interactions that characterized the preceding level; each new structure represented a new set of principles or rules that governed the interaction between organism and environment. One reason the doctrine of stages may have become the focus of attention for developmental psychologists, then, is that it represented a challenge to prevailing empiricist theories, as it implied both the inevitability of the sequence of stages and their resistance to environmental influence.

Stemming from this structuralist theoretical perspective is an inductive research strategy, aimed at inferring the nature of the underlying cognitive system by observing a varied sampling of intellectual behaviours and postulating a model of their underlying mental structure. This strategy implies that any one of these individual behaviours cannot be fully understood and appreciated in isolation. It is only by understanding their relation to each other and to the underlying mental structure they reflect that their true nature can be appreciated.

From the theoretical claim that the cognitive system undergoes a series of major transformations comes a developmental research strategy. The functional rules that describe the interaction between an organism and its environment do not remain constant, as assumed within the empiricist perspective. Rather, these rules undergo transformation, as part of the transformation of the cognitive system as a whole. Each new structure is unique, and consequently the individual at each new stage of development must be studied as a unique organism, different from what it was earlier or what it will be at a later stage of development.

In Piaget's work these postulated structures are represented in the symbolic medium of formal logic, and each of the major structures (sensorimotor, preoperational, concrete operational, and formal operational) is regarded as a broad system of logical operations that mediates, and so unites, a whole range of more specific intellectual behaviours and characteristics. The most appropriate structure to examine as an example of Piagetian stage structures is the structure labelled concrete operations, which allegedly emerges in the age range 6-8, because it has received the most attention both in Piaget's own work and in subsequent research by others.

The central feature that defines the concrete operational thought structure and differentiates it from the earlier preoperational thought structure, Piaget claimed, is the reversibility of mental operations. Mental acts emanating from the preoperational thought structure are irreversible; they cannot be performed in the opposite direction. Thus, judging that A is smaller than B does not entail the identical judgement made from the reference point of B, i.e., that B is larger than A. For this reason, the child conceptualizes phenomena in absolute rather than relative terms. For example, a young child who classifies a ball as *large* is likely to have great difficulty in subsequently regarding this same ball as *small* relative to another, larger ball.

The underlying irreversibility of preoperational thought, Piaget claimed, is what is responsible for many of the unique features of young children's thinking that are described in his investigations. Most central are the absence of operations reflecting the logic of relations, as just illustrated, and the logic of classes, i.e., the ability to conceptualize elements as having multiple membership in a set of hierarchical classes (e.g., living things, human beings, man, father). It is this absence of class logic to which Piaget attributed one of his most widely cited examples of preoperational reasoning: A young child asked if there are more roses or more flowers in a set of 4 roses and 3 tulips is likely to reply more roses. Such a reply, Piaget claimed, reflects the child's inability to simultaneously (and hence reversibly) regard the roses as both a subclass and a part of the larger class (flowers). Hence, the child compares the subclass roses to its complement *tulips*, rather than to the class *flowers*.

The complete system of operations proposed by Piaget as the concrete operational thought structure is an integrated system of reversible operations of classification the combining of elements into groups based on their equivalence; and relation the linking of one element to another in an equivalence relation of symmetry (A is to B as B is to A, as in the case of two brothers), or in a difference relation of asymmetry (A is less than B and B is greater than A). The evolution of this structure was postulated by Piaget to underlie the attainment of conservation also: With concrete operations the child can mentally reverse the transformation (e.g., the pouring of the liquid from the original to a differently shaped container) and hence deduce that the quantity must remain invariant, despite its altered perceptual appearance. In addition, the irreversibility of thought prior to the evolution of the concrete operational structure was alleged to underlie all of the characteristics of young children's thinking that Piaget labeled as "egocentric": the inability to assume the perspective of another, the attribution of one's own psychological characteristics to material objects (animism), and the elevation of the products of one's own psyche (thoughts, dreams) to the status of real, material events visible to others (realism).

Summary

In summary, the constructivist perspective that has just been described and the empiricist perspective described earlier have been the two major theoretical influences leading to the current study of cognitive development. The two perspectives differ from one another on a number of major dimensions. The constructivist views what develops as the internal cognitive system as a whole, the central feature of which is the individual's "meaning making" effort to understand his or her own actions and those of the external world. The empiricist views what develops as independent units of external, observable behaviour, each under the individual control of environmental variables.

With respect to how development occurs, the empiricist posits a cumulative process in which each new behaviour unit is independently acquired through the operation of the same basic mechanism of environmental shaping. The constructivist posits a bidirectional, rather than a unidirectional, interaction between the individual and the environment, leading to a series of major qualitative reorganizations in the cognitive system as a whole, and reflecting progress in the individual's "meaning making" enterprise.

The research strategy employed by the empiricist is a nondevelopmental experimental laboratory strategy devoted to examining the process through which individual behaviour is shaped by environmental contingencies. Empirical investigations are therefore devoted to detailed analyses of a single simple behaviour. The research strategy employed by the constructivist is inductive, as well as developmental. The researcher samples a wide range of behaviours as a basis for hypothesizing the nature of the underlying cognitive system that is presumed to generate these behaviours. Cross-age comparisons are then conducted as a basis for inferring changes that occur in the cognitive system.

It is probably because the two perspectives are so diametrically opposed that the study of cognitive development during the 1960s to a large extent polarized into two camps, with a good deal of the research and theoretical writing during this period directed toward demonstrating the merits of one of the approaches and deficiencies of the other. Since that time, serious weaknesses have become apparent in each of the approaches. As a result, few theorists or researchers studying cognitive development today would classify themselves as adherents of either the empiricist or the constructivist perspectives in the pure forms in which they have been described here. In turn, several new perspectives have evolved and gained adherents; although each of these new perspectives retains certain aspects of empiricism or constructivism, none is in such polar opposition to another as the original constructivist and empiricist views that preceded them. We turn now to the weaknesses that became apparent in the empiricist and constructivist perspectives.

Limits of Empiricism

It has been suggested that researchers who conducted studies of children's learning and memory in the 1950s within the empiricist tradition dominant at the time had no interest in childhood per se, but used children as subjects of convenience to investigate those processes of learning that were the real focus of their interest. Whether this claim is justified or not, a sizeable accumulation of such research supported a conclusion that gained wide acceptance: The basic mechanisms of learning function in an identical way across species and across humans of different ages. A psychology of learning is therefore applicable to children and adequate to explain development.

The Study of Learning

Subsequent research has forced a modification of this basic conclusion. The most influential series of studies by Kendler and Kendler stemmed directly from the discrimination learning paradigm that was prevalent at the time.

Reinforcement is always administered if the response is made in the presence of either of the two top stimuli and is never administered if it is made in the presence of either of the bottom stimuli. This initial "training" phase of the experiment continues until the subject reaches a pre-established criterion of some number of errorless trials, i.e., repeated presentations of the four stimuli during which the subject always makes the response in the presence of a reinforced stimulus and never in the presence of a non-reinforced stimulus. This basic experimental paradigm was employed with diverse subjects, and so the response and the reinforcer themselves might be anything from a lever press and a food pellet in the case of an animal, to verbal responses and reinforcers in the case of a college student.

At this point the training phase of the procedure ends and the test phase begins. The stimuli remain unchanged during the test phase; only the reinforcement contingencies associated with them are different.

Classical empiricist theories of learning yield a clear prediction. The response (or nonresponse) to each stimulus is regarded as an associative bond that is built up as a function of the reinforcement contingencies. When the shift to the test phase occurs, at least some of these bonds must be relearned. The number of bonds that need to be relearned, however, depends on the type of shift.

Kendler compiled substantial evidence confirming this prediction in the case of animals and young human subjects (under 6 years of age). Uncharacteristically, however, they also studied subjects at a range of older age levels, including adulthood. These older subjects performed contrary to the learning theory prediction: For them, the reversal shift was easier to relearn than the extradimensional shift.

The inability of traditional learning theory to account for the performance of older subjects in these experiments led the Kendlers to develop a new, modified theory that they termed "mediation theory." What the older subject is learning in the training phase of the experiment, the

Kendlers proposed, is not a set of discrete associations between stimuli and responses, but a covert (internal) "mediational" response. This covert response mediates, or controls, the overt responses (i.e., responding in the presence of the black stimuli and inhibiting response in the presence of the white stimuli). The Kendlers initially emphasized the verbal nature of these mediating responses, that is, older subjects had learned and applied verbal labels to the stimuli (size, colour; black, white), which they then verbalized to themselves during the experiment. Subsequently, however, the Kendlers broadened their theory somewhat, regarding mediating responses as any covert symbolic responses the subject makes to common features of the stimuli.

If older subjects do indeed make mediational responses during the training phase, then the predicted relative difficulty of the two shifts changes. In the extradimensional shift, not only the overt response, but also the covert mediating response must be relearned (e.g., size rather than color). In the reversal shift, only the overt responses must be relearned (e.g., respond to white, not black). Therefore, the reversal shift should be easier, which was exactly what the Kendlers found for subjects over the age of 5 or 6.

The Kendlers therefore proposed what was in effect a developmental theory of learning. The traditional model of the formation of discrete stimulus response bonds characterizes the learning of children under the age of 5 or 6. At about this age, children develop mediational learning capacity, and at this point the mediational model becomes a more accurate description of the learning process. The historical significance of the Kendlers' formulation of mediation theory is twofold. First, their theory represents a refutation of the behaviourist maxim that claims that the basic learning process functions in an identical way across the life-cycle. The way an individual learns, the Kendlers' work indicates, depends on the individual's developmental level as a result, learning cannot be studied independently from development.

Second, mediation theory represents a departure from the behaviourist maxim that observable behaviour is the only proper object of scientific study, and that it is not fruitful to postulate unobservable internal constructs that mediate this observed behaviour. The Kendlers' work indicates that speculating about internal processes was, in this case, the only route to an adequate conceptualization of the external behaviour that was observed. By not doing so, one ran the risk of serious misinterpretation. In the shift experiments, the achievement of laboratory rats, 5 year-olds, and college students appears equivalent at the end of the training phase (though one group may require more trials to reach the criterion than another). The performances of the respective subject groups during the test phase, however, indicate that the learning that takes place during the training phase although it appears equivalent in its external manifestations is actually quite different across subject groups. A theory that would make reference to the processes underlying these seemingly equivalent observable performances seemed the only way to explain the differences in performance that the subsequent test phase revealed to be present. In other words, the Kendlers' work pointed to the importance of a distinction that would become critical in future work in cognitive psychology: the distinction between product (performance) and the process that generated it.

Study of Memory

Some notable parallels exist between historical developments in the study of learning and historical developments in the study of memory. In this section, some of the latter are summarized and common characteristics are noted.

Memory as Storage. According to the empiricist perspective that dominated psychology in the 1940s and 1950s, learning and memory were but two sides of a single coin. Consider, for example, the paired-associate paradigm discussed earlier. Learning refers to the process by which the associative bond (between the two nonsense syllables) is formed, memory to the retention or storage of that bond, once it has been formed. Because the stimuli are meaningless to the subject, i.e., because the subject has no prior history of associations to them, they were considered as the ideal medium in which to study the basic processes of learning and retention in their pure form. By employing these elementary, "neutral" stimuli, basic properties of the human learning and memory apparatus might be identified. For example, how many exposures are required for an association to be formed and what is the organism's storage capacity for these associations, once they are formed?

Memory as Construction. Memory became a popular research topic in the 1960s, and many laboratory studies were conducted using both children and adults as subjects. The findings from much of this research, however, were difficult to reconcile with the concept of memory as a storage of associations. Consider, for example, memory for an arrangement of chess pieces on a chessboard after a subject studies the board and it is then removed. One might anticipate that studies of this nature would provide indices of the capacity of the human visual memory system. Such estimates, however, have been found to be dependent on the subject's familiarity with the stimulus material and the constraints imposed on the stimulus material to be remembered, that is, whether the pieces are arranged on the board randomly, or in a pattern that conforms to the rules of chess. If the arrangement is random, chess experts and non-chess players show equal memory capacity; if the arrangement is legitimate, however, chess experts display greater memory capacity than non-chess players, even when the chess experts are children and the non-players adults. Thus, one cannot speak of any absolute memory capacity, even one that increases in an age linked manner. It all depends on what is being remembered, relative to the individual's existing knowledge and cognitive system.

A great many other studies have suggested that, when processing a piece of information to be remembered, an individual does not store it in its intact form as an isolated unit. Instead, the individual assimilates the new information to a framework provided by the individual's existing knowledge, often altering or elaborating this new information in a way that is consistent with this existing knowledge base. In a series of studies, Paris and his coworkers asked children simple questions to assess their memory of short narratives. Even young children were willing to reply "yes" to a question such as "Did she use a broom?", when the story stated only, "She swept the kitchen floor". Moreover, by the age of 9 children were able to recall a sentence such as the preceding one from the cue "broom" as effectively as from the cue "swept", even though one had been explicitly and the other only implicitly present.

It would appear, then, that subjects integrate new material into a framework provided by their existing knowledge and draw on this existing knowledge to make inferences that go beyond what is explicitly presented. As a result, newly acquired material cannot be clearly separated from what is already known. Memory, then, is more aptly conceptualized as a process of construction, or reconstruction, than as a process of storage. As such, it cannot be strictly separated from broader processes of reasoning and comprehension, i.e., from the individual's more general "meaning making" activity.

Memory and Development. If memory is part of the broader cognitive system, then developmental changes in this system ought to have implications for memory functions. This has been demonstrated in both a narrow and a broad sense. In the narrow sense, the level of comprehension of material to be remembered should affect how and how well it is remembered. A simple demonstration of this influence has been provided by studies of children's ability to draw an ordered set of sticks of graduated length after they have viewed it and it has been removed. Children who do not comprehend the logic of asymmetrical relations (as revealed by their inability to construct a seriated array from a set of randomly ordered sticks of different lengths) are less able to draw a seriated array from memory after viewing one; rather, they report very different configurations as what they "remember" having seen.

In the broad sense, transformations of the cognitive system ought to affect the memory function itself. Indeed, a wide range of studies indicating such developmental changes have been conducted. The bulk of these studies have centred around the utilization of strategies to enhance memory. Organizing the material to be remembered into conceptual categories and rehearsal, for example, are both strategies that aid memory. Children under the age of Piaget's concrete operational stage show negligible use of these or other strategies to aid memory. For example, given a list of items to memorize containing foods, animals, toys, and items of clothing in a random order, older children and adults tend to recall the individual items within these superordinate categories; young children show no such organisational tendency in their recall. The absence of strategic devices in young children's performance on memory tasks is further substantiated by the finding that young children perform equivalently in a memory task whether they are instructed to try to remember the presented items or simply to look at them. Later, we shall consider further what governs the development and utilization of cognitive strategies such as these. The most important implication to note here is that, as the Kendlers' work demonstrated with respect to learning, memory functions cannot be studied without regard to the subject's developmental status.

Summary

The work described suggests that neither learning nor memory can be studied profitably as a basic process that functions uniformly independent of what it is that is being learned or remembered and its relation to what the learner already knows. Given this, two implications for the study of the development of learning and memory follow, each of which has received considerable empirical support. Developmental change in the cognitive system influences learning and memory performance in the narrow sense that the level of comprehension of new material affects how and how well it is both learned initially and remembered. Developmental change in the cognitive system affects learning and memory in the broad sense that it influences the learning or memory function itself, i.e., the strategies the individual utilizes in executing the task.

Perhaps the most telling indicator of the evolution that has been described is that in contrast to the 1950s and 1960s, few current psychologists classify their work as exclusively devoted to the study of learning or of memory. Rather, they tend to classify themselves as cognitive psychologists, interested in study of the cognitive system as a whole. In some ways, the evolution described might be interpreted as a failure of the principle of reductionism. The principle of reductionism and the related principle of parsimony led to the invocation of a single basic mechanism that accounted for the acquisition of new behaviour, irrespective of the behaviour, the organism, or the relation between the two. The research reviewed here indicates that this assumption is unwarranted. As a research strategy, reductionism dictated that very simple behaviours were to be isolated and studied independently. Once the acquisition mechanism governing these very simple isolated behaviours was understood, an understanding of more complex and significant forms of behaviour would follow. It is fair to say that this promise has not been realized. It is now largely accepted that the search for a single content- and context-free acquisition mechanism will not be fruitful, and that mastery of new cognitive material cannot be investigated isolated from the broader context of the meaning the subject attributes to the material and to the task.

The implications for methodological practice are substantial. In the case of the paired-associate research paradigm strong critics have characterized the studies themselves, not just the task material, as nonsensical and doomed to failure on the grounds that the learning that is observed is of no meaning or relevance to the learner; that is, it occurs completely out of any context, and therefore cannot possibly provide insight into natural context-bound processes of learning. At a minimum, it has been well established that context and meaning have a profound effect on performance. Preschoolers asked to memorize a list of items, for example, on the average remembered only half as many items as they remembered when asked to retrieve a series of items from a make-believe grocery in the next room. Thus, studying the acquisition of arbitrary (meaningless) material in artificial settings offers, at best, limited insight into the acquisition of meaningful material as it occurs in complex, meaning-rich contexts. This limitation has been particularly severe in the study of memory development, in which work has largely been confined to the laboratory study of memory for arbitrary stimuli. As will be noted later, however, the last ten years have seen an increasing concern with the investigation of cognitive functions and their development in contexts (such as Istomina's) that are meaningful to the individuals being studied.

Even a rejection of reductionism, and the resulting theoretical and methodological concepts of a context-free acquisition mechanism, however, does not force a total repudiation of the empiricist view. A few theorists, such as Bijou and Baer, have retained an orthodox behaviourist perspective. More common, however, are the "neo-behaviourist" formulations proposed by the Kendlers and several others. Largely abandoned by the neo-behaviourists are the refusal to speculate about internal processes, reductionism in its radical form, and the nondevelopmental research strategy. Common to all of these neo-behaviourist formulations, however, is the endorsement of the empiricist solution to the question of mechanism: Mind is shaped from without by the unidirectional effects of the environment.

Limits of Constructivism

Empirical evidence incompatible with the theory brought into focus the limitations of orthodox behaviourism as an explanatory framework for cognitive development. During the 1960s and 1970s, American developmental psychologists conducted extensive research related to Piaget's work, much of it disconfirming predictions derived from Piagetian theory. One might have expected, then, that this work, in a similar way, would have brought into focus the limitations of constructivism as an explanatory framework for cognitive development. In this case, however, matters are more complex, for it was not to constructivism that researchers principally addressed their studies, but to Piaget's doctrine of stages.

Stages

The most straightforward prediction derived from stage theory is that the various behaviours that are the alleged manifestations of the underlying stage structure ought to emerge in synchrony, as indicators of the emergence of the underlying structure. In the case of the various behaviours alleged to be manifestations of the concrete operational structure, a large number of studies were performed replicating Piaget's findings that these behaviours emerge between the ages of 6 and 8. Researchers then went on to investigate whether, within individual children, these behaviours appear synchronously at some point during this age period an issue with respect to which Piaget himself had not reported empirical data. A substantial amount of data has now been collected, none of which has yielded strong evidence that concrete operational concepts, such as hierarchical classification, seriation, transitivity, conservation, and various forms of perspective taking, emerge synchronously, even though they all appear during the same general age range.

In the face of these findings, some developmentalists came to Piaget's defense, objecting that Piagetian theory does not proclaim a precisely synchronous emergence of behaviours but rather only their emergence during a period of several years, by the end of which they are consolidated into the structured whole specified by the theory. Others objected to this apparent lack of synchrony on methodological grounds: The set of tasks administered to a subject to assess the various concepts, they claimed, had not been equated with respect to their more superficial performance demands, which had little to do with the concept itself. One assessment task, for example, may have been presented in a manner that made greater demands on the subject's verbal skills than did the other tasks, and for this reason the display of the concept being assessed by this task was delayed relative to the concepts assessed by the other tasks.

This second objection, however, points to what is an even more fundamental problem for stage theory: Even slight, and what one would expect to be insignificant, modifications in task format can drastically alter the likelihood that subjects will exhibit the concept being assessed. For example, whether children will recognize the subclass as part of the class (class inclusion) in the earlier example of roses and flowers is affected by the numerical ratio between the two. Thus, even *within* a single task or concept domain, whether the concept is judged to be present or absent depends to a considerable extent on the particulars of the assessment procedure. The sizeable literature that has accumulated on children's attainment of Piagetian concepts shows this to be the case for every one of the concepts investigated. Using one assessment procedure, for example, 30% of

6- year-olds might be assessed as having attained a particular concrete operational concept. Using a slightly different procedure, perhaps 70% of the same group of 6-year-olds would be assessed as having attained the concept. On what basis does one decide which procedure yields the "true" incidence of attainment?

These demonstrations of so-called task variance were particularly significant because they suggested that Piagetian assessment tasks are not "pure" measures of an underlying reasoning competency, in the way that Piaget's descriptions of them tended to imply. Rather, a number of distinguishable skills appeared to be involved in the successful performance of a task, many of which were not an integral part of the reasoning competency that was the focus of the assessment. Consider, for example, the concept of transitivity, allegedly part of the concrete operational structure. Once the child's mental actions involving relational comparisons of the form A > B are organised into a reversible mental structure, such that A > B is recognised as entailing B < A, Piaget theorized, this reversibility should enable the child to mentally construct a seriated array, i.e., A > B > C > D, as well as to derive additional order relations from those that are given. For example, given A > B and B > C, the child should be able to make the inference A > C. Because it is understood that B participates in dual relationships, one as less than A and another as greater than C, it can serve as the mediator that links A and C. Piaget referred to this inference as the inference of transitivity.

A number of subsequent studies of the transitivity inference, by Trabasso, Bryant and others, aimed to demonstrate that there is more involved in making an inference of transitivity than the inference itself. Each of the individual relations, i.e., A > B and B > C, must first be attended to and encoded by the subject. Each relation must then in some manner be represented and retained in the subject's cognitive system. Failure to achieve any of these steps would be sufficient to prevent the inference from being made, for example if the subject forgot one of the initial relations. The studies by Trabasso and Bryant endeavoured to show that if the successful execution of these initial components were ensured (for example, by exposing subjects to extended training with respect to the initial relations), children several years younger than the ages reported by Piaget showed successful performance on a transitivity task. Similar analyses of other concrete operational concepts have been proposed, for example, Trabasso et al.'s (1978) analysis of the class inclusion concept.

In addition to suggesting that multiple skills enter into performance on a Piagetian reasoning task, the Trabasso and Bryant studies are examples of the numerous so-called "training" studies conducted in the 1960s and 1970s, which will be examined in more detail later, in a discussion of methods for studying developmental change. In these studies, attempts were made to induce a particular concept alleged to be part of the Piagetian stage structure, by exposing children who had not yet attained the concept to some form of training in an experimental laboratory session. Whether the changes from pretest to posttest assessment that occurred in many of these studies were superficial or genuine became the topic of extended debate. At the very least, however, the studies demonstrated that with relatively minimal instruction children could be taught to display some of the behaviours characteristic of the stage structure they had not yet attained naturally, bringing into question the claim that such behaviours are integral parts of a structured whole.

All the forms of evidence described so far evidence of asynchrony in emergence, of heterogeneous skills contributing to performance on assessment tasks, and of the susceptibility of this performance to environmental influences contributed to an increasing disenchantment with the Piagetian doctrine of stages during the 1970s. Positing a single, unified structure, the evolution of which is totally responsible for all of the more specific changes in intellectual functioning that occur over the course of development, appeared an oversimplification that did not accord with a growing body of research data. In a certain sense, stage doctrine in its strongest form appeared to be a kind of reductionism of an opposite sort to that employed by those working within the empiricist framework: Instead of the accumulation of large numbers of individually governed small behavioural units, development could be reduced to the evolution of a single, unitary, all-encompassing structure.

The disenchantment with stage theory was furthered by the fact that Piaget's descriptions of the major stage structures, such as concrete operations, were not closely linked to the actual mental processes in which a subject might engage when responding to one of the typical assessment tasks. Rather, these structures were described in terms of formal logical models that were so abstract and removed from surface behaviour that readers of Piaget's descriptions were left uncertain as to how such models might ever be validated as true portrayals of the individual's mental functions or structure.

In the absence of satisfying answers to these questions, large numbers of developmental psychologists turned away from stage theory, in search of what they hoped would be more promising models of cognitive development. The problem came, however, in articulating a replacement for stage theory. To conclude that the positing of a single, unified structure as what develops is an oversimplification does not dictate the opposite extreme: that discrete competencies develop entirely independent of, and unrelated to, one another. The truth almost certainly lies between these two extremes. The central theoretical and research challenge, then, becomes one of characterizing the interdependencies that exist between developments that occur within distinct domains. Note, however, that the question posed is one about the developmental process: To what extent and in what manner do developmental changes that occur within domains interact with one another as they take place?

In many ways, theorists and researchers in cognitive development were not in a strong position at this point to formulate theoretical models or research hypotheses regarding the developmental process. As we have observed, Piaget's views on developmental process had received relatively little attention from American developmental psychologists in favour of the derivative theory of stages. The tendency in many circles, then, was to discount Piaget's theory in its entirety in rejecting the stage doctrine. On the other hand, there was little enthusiasm, following developmental psychology's absorption with Piaget, for a return to an empiricist conception of mechanism, which had become widely perceived as inadequate.

Constructivism

Questions about structures, it was suggested, are really questions about the process of construction of these structures, and it is understanding of the former that provides a key to conceptualizing the latter. It can be argued that the study of stages within developmental psychology reached a dead end because one cannot study structures independently of the constructive processes that give rise to them. Piaget, however, viewed the constructive process in somewhat the same manner as he did structures, that is, in a very general, abstract form, and to some extent this mode of characterization has given rise to a similar set of problems. The process Piaget described is one in which the individual's own actions on the external world generate feedback that leads to the modification of those actions and their reorganization into new interrelationships with one another. In other words, individuals themselves produce their own development. To many, this conception of developmental change seemed a welcome and desirable alternative to the empiricist view of the individual as the passive recipient of effects produced by the environment.

The efforts of those who undertook to explore Piaget's constructivist model, either theoretically or empirically, however, led to the articulation of two related weaknesses in the model. First, the actions generated by the individual's cognitive system that give rise to change are described by the model in such general, abstract terms that it is not easy to draw on the model in conceptualizing the varieties of more specific, cognitively salient acts the individual engages in and their likely influence on cognitive development. For example, cross-cultural findings indicating that conservation of quantity developed more rapidly in cultures that emphasized certain kinds of experiences were not incongruent with Piaget's model, but the model offered no way of predicting the effects of such specific variations in experience.

The second limitation, closely related to the first, is that in emphasizing the role of the individual's own self-generated actions, the constructivist model neglects the social context in which these actions, and therefore cognitive development, necessarily occur. The constructive process, whatever its precise nature, does not take place in a vacuum. In the course of their everyday experiences, children encounter all sorts of implicit or explicit examples of the higher-level concepts that they themselves will acquire. This does not imply that they internalize these examples in any direct or automatic way. But it is equally unlikely that they systematically ignore them. Indeed, specific evidence is now accumulating to show that children attend to external models of higher-level concepts in a sustained and deliberate manner. The objective, then, must be to understand the specific ways in which the individual's constructive activity utilizes these external data.

Summary: Neo-Constructivist Directions

Piaget's work has had on American developmental psychology from its introduction in the 1950s to the present day. During this period, American researchers collected data suggesting asynchrony in the emergence of stage-related competencies, the contribution of heterogeneous skills to performance on assessment tasks, and the susceptibility of this performance to environmental influence. All of these kinds of evidence contributed to a disillusionment with stage doctrine in its strong form the doctrine that all of cognitive development can be accounted for by the evolution of a single, unitary structure. The lesser attention devoted to Piaget's constructivist hypothesis also revealed a set of serious problems and limitations, however, centering around the effects of specific forms of experience on the individual's cognitive development.

Faced with the limitations they perceived in Piaget's constructivist formulation, a number of developmentalists concerned with questions of process sought ways to modify or to expand on the Piagetian model to take into greater account the specific influence of the environmental context in which development takes place. Fischer, for example, while maintaining many of the central features of Piaget's structuralism, proposed a model in which new cognitive skills are at least initially wedded to the concrete contexts in which they are acquired; they are not the totally general, content-free acquisitions implied by Piaget's theory.

Also to a large extent in reaction to the neglect of social context in Piaget's constructivism, a renewed interest has occurred in developmental theories originating within Soviet psychology, notably those of Luria and Vygotsky. As I indicate later, the Soviet perspective has had a substantial impact in recent years on methodology, as well as theory. In contrast to Piaget, both Luria and Vygotsky emphasized the major role played by the social environment in the development of more advanced forms of mental functioning within the individual. It is the child's first social relations, and in particular the resulting exposure to a language system, that give rise to mental development, according to the Soviet view. In Luria's words: "Children assimilate language a ready-made product of sociohistorical development and use it to analyze, generalize, and encode experience. They name things, denoting them with expressions established earlier in human history, and thus assign things to certain categories and acquire knowledge." The mode of such transmission is social interaction: What start out as interpersonal regulations, e.g., a mother guiding her child in performing a task the child is unable to do alone, gradually become intrapersonal regulations the child becomes capable of regulating his or her own actions to produce the performance, without external guidance. Wertsch has conducted interesting observational studies of this process as it occurs during the course of a mother helping her child do a puzzle.

This view of development is appropriately classified as neo-behaviourist according to the criteria specified earlier development is conceptualized as the product of a unidirectional influence of the environment on the individual. Accordingly, although this view balances Piaget's exclusive focus on the role of individuals in producing their own development by emphasizing the external influences stemming from social interaction, it ignores the complementary part of the individual environment interaction, i.e., the role of the individual: Little attention is given to how children attribute meaning to the social interactions they are involved in, and how this attributed meaning mediates the process by which society affects mind. Descriptions of the shift from interpersonal to intrapersonal regulation in parent child interaction provide an insightful conceptualization of how parents structure their behaviour in efforts to aid the child, but offer little insight into the cognitive processes that enable the child to make use of the adult's input.

Despite the essential factors it highlights, it is thus unlikely that the Soviet view on development would prove a wholly satisfactory substitute for Piaget's constructivism. But it is also unlikely that, for the time being, it will have such an opportunity, for the attention of a large number of researchers in cognitive development has turned in another direction.

8

Information Processing Approach for Development

Introduction

The information-processing approach to the study of cognitive development is not as readily classified as the theoretical perspectives examined up to this point. The major reason is that it is, by the admission of its own adherents, not a comprehensive theory of development, or even of cognition; rather, it is an approach to the study of cognition and, to a lesser extent, its development. Thus, it does not take an explicit position on some of the questions that must be addressed by a theory of cognitive development.

The Computer Metaphor

The origins of the information-processing approach are in cognitive, rather than developmental, psychology. A major impetus for its development was the technological innovation of the modem electronic computer. At the heart of the approach is the concept that the human intellect may function as an information processing system, for which a mechanical information-processing system (i.e., the computer) is a fruitful model. How did this approach attract the attention and enthusiasm of a large number of developmental psychologists so rapidly? It is not difficult to trace the major reasons.

Consider the example of the transitivity inference cited earlier. Piaget attributed the child's ability at the level of concrete operations to infer A < C, given the information A < B and B < C, to the underlying thought structure acquiring the characteristic of reversibility: The operation A < B entailed the reverse operation B > A, and B could thus be regarded as simultaneously greater than A and less than C, thereby serving as the mediator linking A and C. This explanation in terms of underlying logical structure, however, does not identify the specific mental processes by which the child produces a judgement of transitivity in a particular instance. Thus, critics of Piaget's structural approach complained that there was no way ever to prove or disprove the correctness of such models as explanations of the child's behaviour.

Furthermore, researchers studying the transitivity inference identified a number of specific processes that must go into its correct performance, e.g., encoding and retention of the initial relations. From this work it is only a short step to the suggestion that the performance of a cognitive task is made up entirely of the serial execution of a number of individual processes such as these. The computer-inspired information-processing model from cognitive psychology offered a formal model of just such a possibility, for it is by means of such serial execution of operations that a computer functions. The guiding assumption underlying the model is that human cognitive functioning is composed of a set of individual processes that operate sequentially and that are not necessarily governed by the same principles of operation. The information-processing approach can be characterized, then, as one that focuses on these individual processes and the manner in which they operate individually and combine serially to produce the final performance.

What are these individual processes? The major source of influence in defining them has been the information-processing operations executed by a computer. It is thus assumed that information from the environment must be encoded and stored in symbolic representational form. Various processes then operate on the contents of this representation, manipulating and transforming it in ways that create new representations. These processes may be constrained by the fixed processing capacity of the system, and representations may be constrained by a fixed storage capacity. When processing is completed, output is generated in the form of a final performance, or solution to the problem.

A few information-processing psychologists have taken the computer metaphor literally and have attempted to describe the cognitive operations generating a performance by means of a very exact and detailed model that could actually serve as a computer programme for the performance. This approach has the attractive feature of containing a ready test of the model's sufficiency: Does the programme successfully simulate performance on a computer? Klahr and Wallace, for example, developed models of the performance of a number of Piagetian concrete operational tasks using a collection of "condition-action" links termed "productions" as the basic elements of their models. In contrast to the study of "condition action" (or stimulus response) links by behaviourists in the 1950s, the work of information-processing psychologists like Klahr and Wallace is focused squarely on modeling those processes inside the black box that behaviourists sought to bypass. An example of the production system proposed by Klahr and Wallace to produce a transitivity judgment, which illustrates the extremely precise, detailed nature of such a model. Every minute aspect of the process must be represented explicitly or the model will fail to meet the sufficiency criterion. The computer cannot make any decisions that the programme has left unspecified.

Klahr and Wallace's models were criticized as replacing one formalism (i.e., Piaget's models employing symbolic logic) with another; and indeed, following their pioneering effort only a few attempts to construct similar models appeared. A good deal of work followed, however, by researchers who endorsed the general spirit of Klahr and Wallace's approach without casting their models in the form of explicit computer simulations. Interestingly, these researchers continued to employ Piagetian tasks in their work, although they began to include tasks from Piaget's formal operational stage as well as the concrete operational stage.

In an approach advocated by Siegler, for example, the child's performance on a task is described by the "rule" to which that performance conforms. The rule specifies a sequence of acts that are performed in order to execute the task. One test of the adequacy of the rule in characterizing the child's behaviour is the extent to which it predicts performance over a variety of specific task items.

The most widely cited example is Siegler's rule-based model of performance on Piaget's balance scale task. The subject is shown a balance scale on which weights are placed at various distances from the center, and the subject must predict whether one or the other (or neither) side of the scale will go down following the removal of a supporting block. Siegler showed that the performance of 5- and 6-year-old children on such problems conformed to what he termed Rule I, in which only the number of weights is considered: Predict that the side with more weights will go down; if the weights are equal, predict balance. Older children's performance conformed better to Rule II: in the case of equal weights, predict that the side with weights at a greater distance from the fulcrum will go down; or to Rule III, which involved processing both weight and distance information without a consistent rule for integrating them. Not until mid- to late adolescence did a fully correct rule (Rule IV) begin to characterize some subjects' performances (consistent with Piaget's findings on this task). The major virtue of this kind of rule-based model of performance on a cognitive task is its explicit characterization of the sequence of mental operations that the individual allegedly utilizes to execute the task.

A somewhat different approach originated with Pascual-Leone and later Case. At the heart of their work lies what they term the "task analysis" of the operations a subject would have to perform in order to execute a cognitive task. An example is their task analysis of Piaget's isolation of variable task. In one form of the task Piaget asked children and adolescents to experiment with a set of rods that differed on several dimensions (e.g., length, thickness, material) to discover what determined their flexibility. Not until early adolescence, Piaget found, do subjects employ an isolation of variables strategy, i.e., hold the level on all other variables constant while systematically varying the level of one variable to assess its effect. Piaget linked this development to the emergence of the cognitive structure of formal operations.

Based on his task analysis, Case argued that what the subject needs to perform this task is very simple:

> All the subject must do is to identify an object with an extreme position value on the dimension to be tested (e.g., a long stick), then identify an object with an extreme negative value (e.g., a short stick), and then check to see if there is any *other* difference between these two objects that might affect the result of interest (e.g., bending).

The virtues of the information-processing approach for analyzing performance on cognitive tasks are readily apparent, and it is easy to see why the approach was particularly attractive to those developmentalists who had become disillusioned with Piagetian stage theory. In contrast to the Piagetian models of cognitive competence which seemed vague, abstract, removed from specific behaviour, and unverifiable information processing analyses offered explicit, precisely articulated models of the series of cognitive operations a subject actually executed when performing a cognitive task. Less readily apparent, however, were several of the strengths of the constructivist approach that were sacrificed in the adoption of the information-processing approach. The reason this loss was less apparent has to do with what we have already noted with respect to the way American psychologists interpreted Piaget, that is, their focus on the theory of stages at the expense of the theory of constructivism.

A Return to Reductionism

The constructivist and information-processing perspectives differ radically in two respects. One is the information-processing perspective's explicit commitment to reductionism, in contrast to the constructivist perspective's explicit commitment to anti-reductionism, or holism. The other is the focus, within the constructivist perspective, on what has been termed "metacognition," in contrast to its de-emphasis within the information-processing perspective. Let us consider the issue of reductionism first.

The dual respects in which the information-processing approach is committed to reductionism closely parallel the respects in which the behaviourist approach of the 1950s and 1960s was committed to reductionism. First, in a theoretical vein, molar behaviour is regarded as being composed of a number of smaller, individually controlled elements. Second, in a methodological vein, the most fruitful research strategy is considered to be the focus on a particular, well-specified task domain, which, once well understood, will permit generalization to broader (and more significant) domains of behaviour. Piagetian theory and research strategy, of course, are notable, in contrast, for their non-reductionistic perspective individual elements can be properly interpreted only in relation to the whole.

Methodologically, the result has been a series of exceptionally meticulous, detailed analyses of the procedures subjects employ in performing a particular task, ones that serve as pioneering models of the precision to which psychological analyses might aspire. One of the criticisms, however, that has been levelled against these task analyses of specific cognitive tasks pertains to their verifiability. Although closer to observable performance than Piaget's logical models, task analyses by no means constitute a magical key that unlocks the secret of how a correct (or incorrect) performance is produced. How do we know that a particular task analysis is correct? Researchers might collect converging behavioural evidence, such as eye movement patterns or reaction times, that are in accordance with what would be predicted by a given task analysis, but alternative hypotheses always remain possible. Indeed, researchers engaged in task analyses of cognitive tasks have tended to produce as many analyses of the same task, e.g., conservation, as there are analyzers of it. Empirical data have not, as yet, served in the role of *disconfirming* a proposed task analysis.

Another criticism of task analysis and the information-processing approach more generally has been that it limits itself to proposing models of performance on specific tasks and has not integrated those models into a broader theory of human cognitive performance. Adherents of the information-processing approach, on the other hand, defend this omission as a matter of appropriate sequence: Precise models of performance in very specific, restricted domains are alleged to be prerequisites for the formulation of broader, more comprehensive theories. Stated differently, the information-processing psychologist justifies, in the short term at least, sacrificing explanatory breadth for explanatory precision. Here again the parallel to the earlier reductionist research strategy adhered to by behaviourists is clear. And so the debate over reductionism continues, with the information-processing approach assuming the pro-reductionist role.

Theoretically, the concept promoted by the information-processing approach that multiple, largely independent processes are likely to be involved in the performance of a cognitive task has contributed valuably to thinking about cognitive development, particularly as an antidote to Piagetian stage doctrine, which treated performance as the manifestation of a single underlying stage structure. But the problem, and the reductionism debate, arises in deciding whether it is justified to go on to maintain that the performance is nothing but the serial execution of a specified set of individual processes, or whether some higher order organizing entity must be invoked. This brings us to the second major way in which the constructivist and information-processing perspectives differ.

The most serious criticism that has been lodged against the information processing approach is that it has concerned itself predominantly with "strategy execution," and scarcely at all with "strategy selection." In other words, it has largely ignored the processes of "executive" control through which individual strategies are selected, assembled, and monitored. Stated in still different terminology, it has ignored "metacognition."

One can agree with Case that the sequence of strategies he specifies is not difficult to execute, and it is not surprising to learn that he was successful in teaching 8-year-olds to do so. But, if not specifically directed to do so, how would an individual know that this set of strategies ought to be applied to such a problem? Without this knowledge, knowledge of how to execute the strategies is of limited value.

In comparison to knowledge of the first type, i.e., knowledge of how to execute the strategies, which is to a considerable extent ascertainable from the surface features of the performance, knowledge of this second type is subtle and complex. In order to select a strategy as appropriate for solving a particular problem, the individual must understand the strategy, understand the problem, and understand how the strategy and the problem intersect or map onto one another, which entails understanding the range and limits of the strategy's appropriate application. In the case of the isolation of variables strategy this kind of knowledge includes an understanding of: (1) why the isolation or "all other things equal" method is the only means of achieving the task objective; (2) how and why each component of the strategy (such as "... check to see if there is any *other* difference between these two objects that might affect the result") constitutes an essential step in correct application; and (3) why any other strategy would not yield a correct solution.

To be convinced of the importance of this second kind of knowledge, one need only note that it is this knowledge that will determine whether or not an individual utilizes the new strategy when an appropriate situation arises in the natural environment, in the absence of direct instruction. It is the absence of such knowledge that is responsible for the common failures of generalization following training interventions: The subject learns the strategy in the particular context in which it is taught, but fails to apply it subsequently in other contexts in which it is equally appropriate.

Knowledge of one's own cognitive strategy as it applies to a task implies a *reflection* on the strategy that clearly differentiates it from the *execution of* the strategy. The reader may recognize such a developing reflection on one's actions as the heart of the constructivist account of cognitive development that originated with Baldwin and Piaget. It is just this kind of reflection that is involved in strategy selection, to use the language of information processing, but is difficult to incorporate into the information-processing model.

A slightly different aspect of this reflection is implicated in another concept central to Piagetian theory, that of logical necessity. Consider once again the example of the transitivity inference. In the research of Trabasso and his colleagues described earlier, young children who did not show the transitivity concept were trained with respect to each of a set of individual relations, i.e., A < B, B < C, C < D, D < E, using a set of sticks of graduated lengths. It was hypothesized that the subjects encoded and represented the set of relations as a visual image, i.e., A < B < C < D < E. If so, this would explain how a child was able to answer questions about the relation between nonadjacent elements, e.g., A and C, correctly: The child could simply refer to the internal pictorial array that had been formed and produce the information A < C. These findings have prompted an extended debate as to whether these children had indeed mastered the concept of transitivity and Piagetians were quick to make the distinction between an "empirical" judgement of transitivity and a judgement of transitivity that had the characteristic of logical necessity. In other words, the child just indicated might "read off" of her mental representation the fact that A < C, but it does not follow that she sees the relation A < C as an inevitable logical necessity following from the relations A < B and B < C, rather than as an empirical fact that happened to be true but could have been otherwise. This distinction is a difficult one to assess empirically, yet it is this logical necessity of the transitivity judgement that was the heart of the matter for Piaget. And such concepts of logical necessity can only come about as a product of reflection on one's own mental actions, or metacognition—in this case, the mental actions of relating A to B and B to C.

Why is it that those utilizing an information-processing approach tend not to focus on the processes of reflection on one's own cognition that are the core of the constructivist perspective and that are implicated in the concept of logical necessity or the exercise of strategy selection? Rather than an accident, this neglect is most likely ascribable to the fact that the information-processing perspective does not lend itself readily to the incorporation of this aspect of cognition, precisely because its underlying metaphor, the information-processing computer, does not indeed, it cannot reflect on what it is doing at a level differentiated from the "doing" itself. Unlike humans, computers do not "know" what they are doing. The computer can contemplate or evaluate its own actions only in the limited sense represented by the programmemer specifying the operations that will constitute such an "evaluation," e.g., a condition action link directing that processing be terminated once a certain set of conditions is met, but again, these "evaluating" operations are not at a level that is distinct from the processing operations themselves.

Summary: Toward a Developmental Information-Processing Model

It has been attempted here to highlight both the strengths and the limitations of the currently popular information-processing approach to the study of cognitive development. The major strength noted is the explicitness and precision with which it attempts to model specific kinds of cognitive performances. In addition, the information-processing approach is responsible for the concept that performance is composed of a set of sequentially operating individual processes. This specificity and precision, however, is tied closely to a significant limitation the scant attention that has been paid to the integration of specific models into a broader theory of cognition and, particularly, cognitive development.

The major limitation that has been focused on is the lack of attention to what have been termed metacognitive processes. If the information-processing approach is not to restrict its explanation of cognitive development unduly, it will eventually have to go beyond the literal model of the computer to incorporate the reflective, or evaluative, components of cognition and cognitive development. One indication that it is attempting to do just that is the increasing attention that researchers working within the information-processing approach are paying to so-called "executive" strategies. One impetus for this interest has been the frequent finding that subjects are able to execute all of the component strategies that a task analysis deems are required for performance of a certain task, and yet do not assemble those components to produce the performance. Something else appears necessary for success. The term metacognition, as both Brown and Sternberg and Powell note, has been employed very broadly to refer to both the regulation of one's own cognitive processes and knowledge about those cognitive processes. Research pertaining to metacognition thus far has been largely confined to attempts to assess metacognitive knowledge. Is a child aware, for example, that the organization of items into categories is a strategy that is useful to employ to enhance recall? Younger children, we noted, show little awareness of the utility of these types of strategies.

The increasing attention given the topic of metacognition suggests a growing belief in the significant role it is likely to play in understanding cognitive development. What is necessary, however, is a fruitful conceptual and methodological framework in terms of which metacognitive processes can be studied. Despite its centrality in his theory, Piaget's treatment of the topic has proven too abstract and divorced from specific contexts to generate much empirical research. On the other hand, the computer model that underlies the information-processing approach is not well-suited to capture metacognitive processes.

One further limitation of the information-processing approach, only alluded to until now, is one that has been widely noted and acknowledged by both followers and critics of the approach: Information-processing models offer no explanation of change. This limitation is obviously crucial if the approach is to provide an account of development. Why and how is the information-processing system modified over the course of development? However, information processing is in good company here, for it is the mechanism of change that has proven the most difficult and formidable problem for all theories of cognitive development. Let us turn again, then, to the more general question of mechanisms of developmental change.

Mechanisms of Developmental Change

Only a decade or two ago, it appeared as if the question of mechanism in cognitive development was a clear-cut one. There were only two possibilities, and it seemed, moreover, that the data from a set of critical experiments would make it easy to choose between the two. Either the learning theorists were right, and the same basic processes of learning could account for development as well, or Piaget was right and a small number of reorganizations of the cognitive system as a whole that occurred only a few times during the course of the individual's development were sufficient to account for all developmental change.

To decide between these two alternatives, it was thought, one needed only to conduct some so-called "training" studies. In a training study, the investigator attempts to induce via simple learning mechanisms competencies held by Piaget to be manifestations of a global stage structure. If these studies were successful, the developmental process could be explained by simple learning mechanisms. If they were unsuccessful, Piaget's concept of global stage transformation would be implicated.

Remarkably, several hundred training studies were carried out in the decade from the early 1960s to the early 1970s. Even more striking, the vast majority of these studies were devoted to inducing a single Piagetian competency, conservation of quantity. The one thing that can be concluded about these studies is that they did not clearly decide the issue, and "the issue" indeed is now recognized to be much more complex than what we have just portrayed. Many of the studies showed significant changes in children's performance on conservation tasks following training of a variety of different kinds, ranging from telling the children the correct answer ("The amount doesn't change") and rewarding them for making it, to more cognitively oriented attempts to get them to appreciate the logic that dictates the invariance. Exactly what these results implied about how and why children shift during the natural course of development from believing that quantity varies with perceptual rearrangement to believing that it is invariant, however, is far from clear.

In what is perhaps the most widely cited conservation training study, one often praised as a model of elegant experimental design, Gelman claimed that young children fail to conserve because they do not attend to the relevant attribute, e.g., the number of elements rather than the length of the row in the case of number conservation. She demonstrated that by reinforcing children over many trials for choosing as "same" (as a standard) the row with the same number of items but different length (rather than the row of the same length but a different number of items), she could induce many of them to subsequently respond correctly in the standard conservation task, i.e., to respond that the number of items in two rows remained the same after one of them was spread out to be of greater length than the other. In Gelman's terms, she taught such children to discriminate which of two possibilities (spatial magnitude or number) the term "same" refers to. Gelman, however, quite pointedly did not go on to draw from her findings the conclusion that natural attainment of the conservation concept involves "nothing but" (i.e., is reducible to) simple processes of discrimination learning and reinforcement. Nor have the many others who have cited her study been prepared to draw such a conclusion.

Exactly what conclusions ought to be drawn from such studies, then, is far from clear. Much of the uncertainty can be traced to two major sources of ambiguity surrounding experiments that have utilized the training study methodology. First, many observers questioned the validity of the experimentally induced attainments: Had the child merely acquired the surface behaviours indicative of an understanding of conservation or had some genuine change in understanding, i.e., cognitive reorganization, taken place? Although much debate ensued, the matter was largely unresolvable inasmuch as opinion differed widely as to what conservation attainment in fact consists of: Is some underlying cognitive reorganization involved or is it merely the acquisition of a simple empirical fact or rule (quantity doesn't change through perceptual rearrangement)? In others words, what is it that is developing?

Even if these fundamental issues were agreed on, however, and the experimentally induced change were accepted as genuine, a second and even more fundamental and troubling issue remains with respect to the method itself: the issue of *can* versus *does*. If a particular treatment is sufficient to produce a behaviour in an experimental laboratory situation, it does not follow that the salient features of this treatment are always, or ever, involved in the emergence of that behaviour during the natural course of development. It is this second issue that is probably most responsible for the disillusionment that developed with the training study as a tool for investigating mechanisms of developmental change. Perhaps the most striking testimony to its limitations is the fact that despite the 200 or more training studies of conservation conducted in the last two decades, there continues to exist a wide variety of diverse theories regarding the process through which conservation is attained. Thus, the vast conservation training study literature has not significantly constrained theories of the developmental process that underlies the attainment of conservation.

Multiple Dimensions and Mechanisms of Change

Along with the abandonment of the idea of training studies as providing a critical test of empiricist versus constructivist explanations of change came a gradual abandonment of the idea that either view could provide a comprehensive theoretical account of developmental change in cognitive functioning. One reason is that, following in part from work done within the information-processing approach, a considerably more complex picture of what it is that is developing has emerged a "what" that encompasses a diverse set of competencies, rather than only a single entity. As a result, it is likely to require a more complex process, or set of processes, to explain that development. A range of possibilities exists with respect to what it is that may develop, including basic processing capacity, processing efficiency, processes of encoding and representation, strategy possession and execution, and metacognitive processes of strategy selection and regulation. Developmental changes in each of these could conceivably be governed by different mechanisms; moreover, changes in some (e.g., processing capacity) might be invoked to account for changes in others (e.g., strategy usage).

Processing Capacity. A possibility that is very attractive because of its simplicity is that the change responsible for most, if not all, advances in cognitive functioning with age is an increase in basic processing capacity, presumably as the result of neurological development. Thus, this alternative attributes cognitive development most directly to an underlying biological process of maturation. Pascual-Leone has advanced an elaborate "neo-Piagetian" theory of cognitive development founded on the assumption of age-linked increases in absolute processing capacity. The fact that performance increases with age on tests of basic processing such as digit span appears to support such a view. A 3 year-old can repeat an average of only 3 digits, while a 10-year-old can repeat an average of 6 digits.

That such improvements in performance are attributable to increases in processing capacity, however, is extremely difficult, if not impossible, to prove, since a number of hard-to-discount alternative explanations exist. In the instance of digit span, for example, the older child may be employing some strategic device, such as rehearsal or chunking, that the younger child is not. In other words, it is difficult to prove that children of the two ages are executing the task in exactly the same way, the only difference being that the older children have a quantitatively greater capacity. Furthermore, as discussed earlier, capacity is highly influenced by familiarity with the material: If the domain is one in which a young child is highly experienced (e.g., chess boards), that child's recall performance may exceed that of much older children less familiar with the domain. Similarly, Case and his colleagues demonstrated that the capacity of adults drops to that of 6-year-olds if adults are required to execute a digit memory task using a newly learned set of digit symbols.

Processing Efficiency. Case (in press), in opposition to Pascual-Leone, has argued that improvements with age in performance on tests such as digit span only appear to be the result of an absolute capacity increase. Actually, he claims, improved performance is ascribable to an increase in the efficiency with which basic operations, such as encoding, are executed; accordingly, less capacity is required for their execution. This leaves the individual with a greater remaining "functional" capacity for holding the products of those operations in memory, even though the total capacity remains unchanged. In support of his perspective, Case cites recent evidence that performance on measures of basic operations (e.g., counting an array of objects) becomes faster and more efficient with age, making plausible his view that increases in efficiency are at least in part responsible for increases in functional capacity, and hence in performance on processing tests such as digit span. Whether the fundamental change is one of processing efficiency, as Case claims, or of total processing capacity, as Pascual-Leone claims, both believe that this change is itself a function of underlying neurological development.

The issue even more critical to debate, however, is the extent to which age related increases in processing capacity (whether absolute or only "functional") underlie all forms of developmental change in cognitive functioning, as both Case and Pascual-Leone claim. The fact that performance on measures of basic processing improves with age has already been established, as indicated above. But we also know that cognitive functioning changes developmentally in many other ways. Children acquire new, qualitatively different strategies they did not have previously; they integrate existing strategies in new ways; they encode new and different kinds of information and represent it in new and different ways; and they develop new forms of executive, or metacognitive, control over their cognitive functioning. Most developmentalists today would agree with the view that increases in basic processing efficiency and/or capacity are implicated at most as necessary conditions for many of these other kinds of changes. They fall far short of being by themselves sufficient to explain how these changes come about. Let us turn, then, to these other kinds of changes and the mechanisms that may underlie them.

Encoding and Representation. Another factor that undergoes developmental change, and might account for improvements in performance on many kinds of cognitive tasks, is improved encoding and representation of information essential to successful execution of the task. No matter how efficiently they are developed, operations cannot be performed on material that has not been attended to, encoded, and in some manner represented within the cognitive system. Siegler and Klahr emphasize this point nicely in the case of the balance scale task described earlier: At a certain level children encode information about weight but do not encode information about the distance of the weight from the fulcrum, as evidenced by their ability to reproduce weight but not distance information in tests of recall. The encoding of distance information is an obvious prerequisite to the execution of the more advanced strategies in which distance is taken into account, though Siegler's work does not prove that it is a change in encoding behaviour that causes the change in strategy. Conceivably, the causal relationship is in some sense the reverse: The child's intent to use a new strategy leads the child to encode new kinds of information.

Strategy Execution. Through what process does an individual come to use new or modified strategies in performing a cognitive task? Constructivist accounts have traditionally emphasized the role of self-regulatory mechanisms within the individual: The individual gradually constructs a more adequate, comprehensive, and better equilibrated set of cognitive operations to be applied to the external world. But, as noted, these accounts have tended to minimize the role of the external environment. Within some versions of the constructivist account, exposure to material reflecting the higher-level structure toward which the individual is developing is a necessary condition for change, while others theorizing within the constructivist framework hold to the more radical position (reflected in Piaget's writings) that the individual literally constructs anew each more advanced mode of cognitive functioning based on the discrepant feedback produced by actions executed at the existing level. According to this formulation, then, the functioning of the cognitive system leads to its modification, a view endorsed by theorists operating from such disparate frameworks as Piaget and Klahr and Wallace.

This stronger version of constructivism ignores the fact that models of the more advanced concepts or strategies the individual will acquire are often prevalent in the individual's environment, as emphasized by the Soviet theories of Luria and Vygotsky mentioned earlier. Case's work on the isolation of variables strategy suggests that an individual can be taught to execute this strategy through social facilitation, at least in a laboratory context. The role of social influence in its acquisition in natural contexts is another question. But the role of both of these processes (individual construction and social facilitation) must be considered in positing an explanation of how an individual acquires a new strategy. Even though external models are not directly or automatically internalized, it is most unlikely that they are systematically ignored.

Strategy Selection and Regulation. With respect to one final factor, namely the individual's metacognitive decision to utilize particular strategies, the power of social facilitation is less clear. An individual might be instructed successfully in exactly how to execute a particular strategy and even be instructed regarding the conditions under which it is appropriate to apply the strategy, provided these conditions can be well specified. But whether the individual will choose to use the strategy in contexts that are not identical to the one instructed is more problematic. For example, children might be taught to use rehearsal to facilitate memory and yet not employ the strategy in their own activities, a finding that has, in fact, been reported by Paris and Lindauer. As suggested earlier, whether a strategy is selected in noninstructed, natural contexts is likely to depend on individuals' metacognitive understanding of the strategy itself, i.e., their understanding of their own actions. In other words, the individual must understand the value and significance of the strategy as well as how to execute it; and the acquisition of this appreciation, or metacognitive understanding, is likely to be the more difficult, complex attainment of the two.

Piaget proposed that the mechanism underlying the development of both strategies and metacognitive strategies was *equilibration*, the functioning of which he described only in rather general and formal terms. Strategies become consolidated and coordinated with one another through exercise. The feedback from this exercise, however, causes the individual to perceive the limitations of these strategies and provides the impetus, or disequilibrium, necessary for the construction of new strategies that will be more adequate for dealing with the tasks encountered and so leave the organism in a state of improved equilibrium with its environment. Several information-processing theorists have undertaken to introduce a developmental mechanism into their models by describing this kind of process in the language of information processing. Klahr and Wallace, for example, talk about a self-modifying production system with features such as consistency detectors, which lead strategies to become more efficient. Case likewise describes a process whereby a set of strategies becomes modified during the course of their own functioning. Thus far, however, these efforts have not gone beyond the description of the general features of the process, in language that is very different from Piaget's. What would be most useful now are models that would generate new, testable hypotheses about how the process operates.

Summary: New Approaches to Studying Change

Two major factors that have limited progress in understanding the mechanisms of developmental change have been discussed. One is the lack of satisfactory methods of empirical investigation. The other is the scarcity of specific hypotheses that are amenable to empirical test. On the positive side, we now have a considerably more sophisticated conception of what it is that is developing and of the mechanism or more likely mechanisms that will be necessary to account for this development.

Also on the positive side is the fact that in recent years, after being diverted by a number of subsidiary issues, such as the existence of stages, modem developmentalists of virtually every theoretical orientation have identified a better understanding of the process of change as their primary objective, and a great many of them have begun to focus their research efforts on investigating the mechanisms of developmental change. In particular, researchers interested in both learning and development have begun to explore the use of new "microgenetic" methods as a means of obtaining detailed observations of the change process as it occurs. These methods differ markedly from the classical training study methodology discussed earlier, in that the focus is on the change process itself rather than on a comparison of pretest and posttest performance.

Microgenetic methods show promise in affording insight into the change process, though the approaches used do not fit into traditional categories of research methods. Lawler, for example, observed a single subject over several months, during the course of which the child mastered some elementary mathematical concepts. His observations led him to emphasize as a central feature of the developmental process the integration of strategic knowledge that initially functions within isolated, unintegrated domains. Similarly, Kuhn and Phelps observed preadolescent subjects in repeated encounters with a problem-solving task over a period of months. Most subjects' progress, they found, occurred only very gradually and involved the prolonged use of both less and more advanced strategies in conjunction with one another. It was during this period of observation, Kuhn and Phelps proposed, that the subject was gaining metacognitive understanding of which strategies were effective and why, as well as gaining practice in the execution of the more advanced strategies. Their observations also pointed to an aspect of the change process that has been largely ignored. The most formidable problem for subjects appeared to be not the acquisition and consolidation of new strategies but the ability to abandon old, less adequate strategies, which is a reversal of the way development has typically been conceived. Other current approaches to the microgenetic study of developmental change are reflected in work by Feldman within a constructivist framework, and in work by Paris and his colleagues within an information-processing framework; the work by Paris also points to the importance of the metacognitive regulation of strategy usage.

Past-Progress and Future Directions

Psychology over a period of almost half a century, culminating in the current focus on gaining better understanding of the mechanisms of developmental change.

Evolution in Theory

One way to summarize this evolution is as the successive rejection of a series of explanatory mechanisms on the grounds that they are too simple to explain what a theory of cognitive development must account for in other words, the study of cognitive development: How do mind and reality come to be coordinated with one another?

A biologically governed unfolding of developmental forms without regard to environmental influence is no longer taken seriously as a model of psychological development. The more recent hypothesis of a biologically governed, quantitatively increasing processing capacity has similarly been criticized as inadequate to explain how and why cognitive development occurs.

Also rejected as too simple to account for the complexity of cognitive functioning and its development are explanatory mechanisms that bypass the internal functioning that takes place within the organism. Influences of external variables on the developmental process are now widely accepted as mediated by characteristics internal to the individual. Likewise rejected are simple acquisition mechanisms that are purported to function in an identical manner irrespective of the material being acquired and its relation to what is already known by the acquirer and to the capabilities of his or her cognitive system. Put another way, it is now widely accepted that mechanisms of learning and retention do not function independently of the individual's intellect as a whole. Existing conceptual structure provides the basis for the interpretation of new information.Although the individual's intelligence, or active structuring of experience, is thus recognized, there has also been criticism and widespread rejection of explanatory mechanisms that attribute cognitive development to the progressive restructuring of this intelligence as an activity of the individual that takes place isolated from social contexts that might influence it. Individuals develop within a social context of other individuals, and the interdependence of cognitive and social processes must therefore be acknowledged and investigated.Parallel with this evolution in the concepts of an adequate explanation of developmental process has been an evolution in concepts of what it is that is developing. The concept of isolated competencies that accumulate independently has been rejected for ignoring the crucial organizational features of behaviour and knowledge. But the concept of a single, structured whole that develops as an integrated entity and mediates all more specific components of cognitive functioning has also been rejected. A major contribution of the information-processing approach has been to highlight the fact that there exist a number of distinct cognitive functions, each of which may undergo developmental change. A unique contribution of the constructivist perspective, on the other hand, and one difficult for the information-processing approach to encompass, is its focus on what is now termed metacognition and its development in other words, the individual's reflection on his or her actions and the "meaning making" endeavor that this reflection is a part of.The preceding summary conversely serves to prescribe the features a fully satisfactory explanatory account of cognitive development would need to possess:

1. It would need to refer to the mental processes that take place within the organism, including those processes termed metacognitive.
2. It would need to characterize development as a gradual coordination of individual mind and external physical and social reality, in which neither internal nor external forces predominate over the other.
3. It would need to address the social contexts in which development occurs and the ways in which those contexts relate to individual development.
4. It would need to account for context specificity of cognitive attainments as well as transsituational commonalities in cognitive functioning.

5. It would need to specify the mechanisms by which developmental change occurs.

During the next several decades, theories that are proposed to account for cognitive development are likely to possess at least the preceding characteristics, as well as others not yet clear. That this is so serves as an indication that the field has progressed, despite the absence of an accumulation of the "hard facts" a reader of this chapter might have anticipated.

Evolution in Method

Not surprisingly, as the field of cognitive development has evolved in its theoretical sophistication, so it has also evolved with respect to its methods, and this latter evolution also gives reason for optimism regarding the field's future. A decade or so ago, researchers in the field of cognitive development could be portrayed, with some justification, as preoccupied with a narrow range of cognitive phenomena investigated in experimental laboratory contexts, where both phenomenon and context were of uncertain relevance to children's cognitive functioning and development in natural settings. Meanwhile, crucial practical decisions as to how children might be reared and educated so as to maximize their cognitive potential and their productivity and fulfilment as adults were left to others outside the academic enterprise of cognitive development.

Today, these characterizations of the field of cognitive development are much less accurate than they were. As we have indicated, recognition of the profound effect that context and meaning have on performance has grown, and more and more researchers are undertaking to examine cognitive functioning within the natural contexts of meaningful activities that children engage in school as well as in non-school environments. Cognitive abilities such as reading are currently of great interest to cognitive and developmental psychologists to a large extent because of, rather than despite, their practical importance.

One impetus for this research trend has been the work on cognition and culture by Cole, Scribner and others, work that has been inspired to a large extent by the "contextualist" theoretical perspective of Vygotsky and Luria. A number of cross-cultural investigations have shown that non-schooled populations do poorly on Western IQ test items, which are of course closely related to the kinds of activities engaged in in school. This finding is, by itself, trivial and uninterpretable and highlights the necessity of examining cognition and cognitive development in the context of those cognitive activities that are meaningful and salient in the lives of the individuals being investigated, if meaningful conclusions are to be drawn. The appropriate unit of investigation, it has been suggested, should become cultural practices, not psychological tests and experiments.

This point is equally applicable to research within our own culture. The study of cognitive development in contexts that are not clearly linked to contexts in which cognitive development occurs naturally seriously constrains the insight this study can yield. There are signs that developmental researchers are beginning to take this admonition seriously, and that future academic study of cognitive development will not be as divorced from practical or "applied" concerns as it has been.

This issue of "ecological validity" has been highlighted even further by another trend of the last decade: The study of cognitive development is no longer limited to an exclusive focus on the childhood years. There are indications that it may be fruitful to conceptualize cognitive functioning in adulthood particularly the substantial individual variation in cognitive functioning among adults from a developmental perspective. Parallel to what has been recognized to be the case in cross-cultural work, however, it is apparent that it will be essential to study cognitive functioning beyond the childhood years in contexts that are meaningful and salient to the individuals studied, if our interpretations are to be meaningful.

This expansion of the traditional child-focused study of development to encompass the latter 80% of the life-span promises benefits not only for our understanding of adult cognition, but for our understanding of cognition and cognitive development during childhood as well. The process of cognitive development during childhood can be fully appreciated only to the extent that we understand the end points toward which it is evolving.

The psychoanalysts and cognitive developmentalists, for example, have emphasized the covert relationships between emotional states and behaviour, whereas the ethological-adaptational and social cognitive theorists have focused on the communicative functions of emotional expressions.

Curiously, there has been considerably less disagreement about the central question to be addressed in research and theorizing concerning social development than regarding emotional development. In this area, the principal concern has always been with the mechanisms underlying the formation of enduring emotional bonds or relationships to specific people, notably parents, and the effects of varying social experiences on later personality. However, the major theorists have attempted to provide somewhat different types of explanations, ranging from descriptions to explanations that focus on proximal causes and mechanisms to explanations that dwell on ultimate causes. Nevertheless, a consensus has emerged in the last decade, thanks to the pioneering work of John Bowlby, who brought the perspective of evolutionary biology to bear on social and emotional aspects of early human development.

Major Theories and Approaches

Although many theorists and developmentalists have pondered the nature of socioemotional development, most have provided explanations that can be categorized into one of five major theoretical approaches. In this section, I describe only major theorists characteristic of each approach in an attempt to illustrate the nature of these diverse perspectives.

Psychoanalysis and Its Derivatives

Systematic attention to social and emotional development in infancy began with Sigmund Freud's construction of psychoanalytic theory in the first decade of the twentieth century. Freud's work was of seminal importance for two reasons. First, he was the first theorist to speculate about the formative significance of those early experiences such as feeding, infantile sexuality, and toilet training, which had formerly been considered relatively unimportant. Second, Freud was perhaps the first theorist to pose questions about the development of emotions, rather than about their nature and significance in adults.

Freud proposed that the human mind was organized into three mental systems the id, ego, and superego.

The superego, which governs the moral and ethical conduct of the individual, develops in early to middle childhood and is thus not a factor in infant development.

By contrast, the interplay between the id and the ego is critically important to psychoanalytic theorizing about infancy. Freud viewed the id, which strives for immediate gratification by any available means, as the source of all human motivation.

Unlike the id, which is present at birth, the ego develops slowly and attempts to establish control over the id by ensuring that gratification is obtained only at appropriate times and places. Among the crucial psychological functions of the ego are: the delay of gratification; perception, thought, and language; and the experience and expression of emotions (external expressions) and affects (internal feeling states). The development of the ego can thus be assessed by observing the emergence of these three general functions.

Throughout most of his life, Freud focused on the development of the superego; his concern with infancy and thus with ego development, was one that crystalized only in the last few years of his life. As a result, most psychoanalytic theory concerning early social and emotional development is attributable to Freud's followers, notably Anna Freud (his daughter) and Rene Spitz.

It was Spitz who proposed that ego development is not simply a function of biological maturation; instead, he argued, the emergence of ego processes is primarily determined by the quality of mother-infant interaction. In Spitz's view the major milestones of socioemotional development were "organizers" that reflected the attainment of a new stage of ego development. When maternal care was adequate, biological maturation ensured that these milestones occurred at a predictable time; but when the infant's care was deficient, ego development was retarded and thus the milestones were attained more slowly, if at all.

Psychoanalysts link the major milestones in socioemotional development to ego development, which, in their view, is affected by mother-child interaction, separation, and the child's perception of the mother's physical and emotional accessibility or inaccessibility. According to the psychoanalysts, mother-infant interaction is related to affect development in two ways. First, the mother as primary caretaker assures gratification of the infant's physical needs and this in itself guarantees formative importance. Second, she must often frustrate the child in order to facilitate its integration into society. These frustrations begin early with attempts to train the child to sleep through the night and to feed on schedule. By being the source of both gratification and frustration, the mother is thus responsible for both increases and decreases in drive. Because drive increases produce displeasure, while drive reductions produce quiescence (absence of unpleasure) or pleasure, the mother is inextricably tied into the infant's affective life.

The affects that result from need gratification help to organize the ego processes of perception, cognition, and memory. They facilitate perception by giving salience to stimuli in the environment that coincide with need and need reduction. When mother-infant interaction is generally gratifying, the stimuli that become salient are likely to be those that relate to the mother, particularly her face.

Learning Theory

Shortly after the psychoanalytic movement was launched by Freud in United States. It was founded by John Watson, who was frustrated by the tendency, especially on the part of European theorists, to speculate about the effects of unobservable events or unobservable mental structures and processes. If psychology was to be a science, argued Watson, it must limit itself to phenomena that are empirically verifiable. Impressed by Pavlov's then recent research on classical conditioning in dogs, Watson proposed that emotional development proceeded as a result of learned associations with, or modifications of, one of the three basic (i.e., unlearned or innate) emotions he posited: fear (elicited by loud noises or the loss of support), rage (elicited by the restriction of bodily movements), and love (elicited by stroking, patting, or stimulating an erogenous zone).

Watson's major empirical contribution was the demonstration that fears could be developed through classical conditioning and could be eliminated in the same way. Watson and Rayner, for example, by associating the appearance of a rat with the loud fear-eliciting sound of a gong produced a conditioned fear of rats (and, indeed of all white, furry things). Watson assumed that the same process must underlie all conditioned emotions, not only fears. For Watson, and the learning theorists who followed him, only emotional expressions were of interest; internal affective states were not independently explorable or verifiable and were thus to be ignored.

While classical conditioning aims to account for the transfer of an already existing response to new stimuli that did not initially elicit the reaction, operant conditioning is useful for explaining increases or decreases in the frequency of emotional reactions that occur spontaneously. The operant conditioning of emotional reactions in infants only became the focus of attention in the 1950s, several decades after the learning theory approach was promoted by Watson. Researchers such as Rheingold, Gewirtz, and Ross, Brackbill and Gewirtz showed that rates of smiling, vocalizing, and crying could be experimentally manipulated by the discriminating application of rewards or punishments. A further development of this general approach took place a decade later, when Bandura and Walters reintroduced the notion of learning through mere observation, which they called observational learning. They argued that many behaviour patterns, including emotional expression, could be learned simply by seeing them displayed by other people. However, they did not explicitly consider infant emotional behaviour.

Ethological-Adaptational Theory

Unlike psychoanalysts and learning theorists, ethological-adaptational theorists such as Bowlby consider the communicative functions of emotions to be of paramount importance. As a result, they tend to focus on why people perceive emotions and experience affects, and what purpose emotions and social relationships serve. During infancy, they argue, emotional expressions such as smiles and cries affect the behaviour of parents and caretakers and thus play a special role in regulating social relationships. More specifically, Bowlby proposed that these signals promote proximity to protective adults, and thus would have had great survival value in the environment in which humans originally evolved.

Bowlby went further, suggesting that the repeated association of proximity promoting signals with appropriate (i.e., proximity-promoting) responses on the part of adults underlies the formation of attachment bonds between infants and adults. In so doing, Bowlby not only provided an answer to questions about why emotions and social relationships exist in infancy (they exist because they have survival value), but also proposed a mechanism whereby social bonding might proceed. Bowlby, who was trained as a psychoanalyst, believed that his theory, based on the principles of modem evolutionary biology, provided a more defensible model of emotional dynamics than did Freud's notion that emotional energy was regulated by the hypothetical mental structures, id, ego, and superego.

Cognitive-Developmental Approaches

While recognizing the potential function of emotional states and expressions, another group of theorists has, since the 1940s, been concerned with the cognitive processes that are the proximate causes of emotions or affects. In a seminal contribution, Hebb sought to explain how fear came to be elicited by the appearance of a novel stimulus one that by definition could not have been associated with unpleasant consequences because it had never been encountered before. Hebb provided a physiological explanation in terms of the discrepancy between the pattern of stimulation occasioned by previous encounters with familiar stimuli and the stimulation produced by the novel stimulus. This discrepancy produces the distress which we call fear, Hebb argued. Modifying Hebb's formulation, developmental psychologists such as Kagan and McCall provided an explanation of the same sort, in which they attributed fear or distress to the discrepancy between memories (or schemata) and the features of novel objects.

In terms of the discrepancy model, the magnitude of an emotional response varies depending on the degree of similarity between the novel stimulus and the schemata to which it is compared. When there is great similarity, there is little discrepancy, and thus little distress is occasioned. As the magnitude of the discrepancy increases, the amount of distress increases, up to the point at which discrepancy becomes so great that the stimulus cannot be assimilated. The amount of distress thereupon starts to decrease producing an inverted U-shaped curve relating distress to degree of discrepancy. Kagan has argued that the discrepancy model can account for emotional phenomena such as smiling, separation anxiety, and stranger anxiety or wariness.

Social Cognition

The most recent perspective to gain prominence is the social-cognitive approach. There is really no unified theory here, but an approach which like the cognitive-developmental theory—emphasizes the infant's attempts to make sense of or interpret its experiences. Many of those who take this perspective have attempted to make their perspective an adjunct to Bowlby's ethological-adaptational theory.

Despite similarities with the cognitive developmentalists, those who have proposed a social-cognitive approach differ in important ways from them. Where the cognitive developmentalists focus on discrepancy, one group of social-cognitive theorists has emphasized ambiguity, and has emphasized the communicative function of emotional expressions. For example, Campos and his colleagues have shown that when in ambiguous situations, infants of 10 months of age and older will examine their mothers' faces for emotional cues presumably because this information may help them to disambiguate the situation. The child then modifies its emotion and behaviour in accordance with the mother's emotional expression.

The propensity to both seek and utilize the information thus obtained may vary depending on the degree of trust the infants have in their mothers. The development of trustful relationships has itself been an issue of concern to social cognitive theorists. Following Ainsworth, Lamb has suggested that variations in the responsiveness and sensitivity of parents to their children's signals may produce differences in the extent to which children come to count on their parents' reliability, consistency, and appropriateness of response.

Summary

The approaches, emphasis, and assumptions are remarkably different. Notice, however, that each group has asked a slightly different question. Psychoanalysts have focused on the way in which social experiences retard or accelerate the endogenous processes underlying development. Learning theorists have focused on the way in which social experiences affect the emergence or later development of certain emotional reactions in the absence of any underlying endogenous developmental process. The ethological adaptational theorists have asked what purpose these emotional reactions might currently serve or might have served during the evolutionary history of the species. The cognitive-developmental theorists have asked what basic cognitive processes underlie changes in social and emotional behaviour, while those who adopt a social-cognitive perspective propose that we may obtain a broader view of socioemotional development if we assume that children actively try to make sense of, or to understand, their social and nonsocial experiences.

Thus we find both differences in basic assumptions and differences in focus. This means that while perspectives which make incompatible assumptions are obviously inconsistent with one another (e.g., psychoanalysis and learning theory), the others may all contribute something to our understanding of socioemotional development, with the joint insights being more useful than those provided by any one approach on its own.

Milestones in Socioemotional Development

Despite great differences in approach and emphasis, all of the approaches described above have attempted to explain a narrow set of social and emotional phenomena. As far as emotional development is concerned, focus has fallen on the emergence of social smiling, fearful reactions to strangers, and distressed reactions to separation from the parents. The major milestone in social development is the formation of discriminating social attachments, which is, in most accounts, temporally linked to the emergence of separation anxiety. In this section, nature of these five milestones, and then in the next section, discuss the way in which each group of theorists has attempted to explain these aspects of emotional development.

Social Smiling

Although newborns and even preterm infants produce facial expressions that resemble smiling, these expressions usually occur when the infant is either drowsy or sleeping, and seem to represent involuntary physiological reactions. Voluntary smiling (e.g., smiles elicited by social bids from adults) in a waking state usually does not occur until the infant is 4 to 6 weeks of age. Initially, smiles are elicited by a variety of stimuli, including faces, bells, and bull's-eyes but gradually they are limited to social stimuli and contexts, with the human face, viewed full-on, becoming the most effective stimulus for eliciting smiles. At first, the eyes appear to be most important, as a stimulus containing little more than two dots is effective in eliciting smiles. Over time, however, the infant comes to require a richer, more facelike stimulus if smiles are to be elicited. From the second and third months, the infant appears capable of recognizing specific faces, and thereafter, the faces of familiar people such as family members and perhaps regular babysitters elicit smiles most readily. Less familiar individuals elicit weaker smiles and must work harder to elicit any.

Stranger Anxiety or Wariness

Although positive reactions to strange adults are somewhat muted from late in the first quarter year, frankly negative reactions typically do not occur until the third quarter year of life. The intensity of these reactions varies from infant to infant: Some infants may only sober when they encounter a stranger, whereas others may cry intensely and retreat rapidly. Initially called "eight month anxiety" because Spitz believed that these reactions predictably emerged at eight months, it has now become clear that the onset of negative stranger reactions is highly variable from one infant to the next, although all infants seem to pass through a phase of adverse responses to strangers, usually beginning between 6 and 15 months of age. One group of researchers reported a second peak around 18 months, but this is not well established. Situational characteristics also affect the intensity of stranger reactions, as Rheingold and Eckerman and Sroufe, Waters, and Matas have shown. Specifically, the intrusiveness and strangeness of the adult's behaviour, as well as the proximity and accessibility of the parent, and the familiarity of the location, all affect the intensity of distress or wariness. In many cases, signs of wariness, distress, or avoidance alternate with indices of positive affiliation, indicating that infants are often attracted to strangers as well as alarmed by them.

Separation Anxiety

When distress occurs following separation from parents in infants under 6-8 months of age, it appears related to the termination of enjoyable activities; infants are readily mollified by substitutes who take up where the departing person leaves off. Hereafter, however, distress appears related to separation from specific persons, and children are often dissatisfied with substitutes. If the separation is prolonged, the reaction changes from distress, agitation, and anger (termed protest) to despondency and apparent depression (called despair), to apparent recovery (otherwise known as detachment) as the child regains responsiveness to social overtures. Long-term separations that take place prior to the onset of separation anxiety around 6-8 months (as, for example, when a child is moved from a foster home to an adoptive home) may produce temporary disequilibrium as the child adjusts to new routines and styles, but there is no comparison with the intensity of protest and despair observed when older infants experience the same separations.

Social Attachments

The emergence of discriminating separation protests is usually viewed as evidence that children have formed specific attachment bonds to the person concerned. Other indices of these bonds include: Use of the adult as a 'secure base,' whose presence facilitates exploration; selective use of the adult for comfort or protection in the event of distress or fear; and a preferential desire for proximity to, or contact with, the adult.

As mentioned earlier, infants begin to show preferences for familiar over unfamiliar adults from the first quarter-year of life. Although they are clearly part of the process leading up to attachment, theorists have been unwilling to describe these early preferences as indices of attachment. Most theorists believe that the emergence of separation protest signals a major qualitative change in the nature of social relationships. For the first time, the child reacts differentially to the absence of a person, rather than simply to his or her presence. This suggests a change in the child's cognitive capacity perhaps the onset of recall memory or object permanence which allow the child to remember, and therefore miss, the parent when he/she is not present. This qualitative change, manifest behaviourally by the emergence of separation anxiety, is often viewed as a sign that true social attachments to specific individuals have been formed.

Fear of Heights

The second half year of life is noted not only for the emergence of fear of strangers and separation anxiety; it is also a time when several nonsocial emotional changes take place.

The best studied of these is the emergence of a fear of heights, even though psychologists have only in the last decade come to recognize that the fear of heights is as much an aspect of emotional, as of perceptual, development. Because some animals appear fearful on the deep side of the visual cliff from birth or from the time they are able to see, many had speculated that the fear of heights was innate. This does not appear to be the case in humans. The first crucial study was one by Campos, Langer and Krowitz in which it was shown that by 2-3 months of age infants could distinguish between deep and shallow drop-offs when suspended over them: their heart rate predictably decreased when they viewed depth, indicating attention and interest. Later Fox, Aslin, Shea, and Dumais used a more complex procedure to show that the stereoptic perception of depth emerged around 3-4 months. Interestingly, however, infants of this age do not show any signs of fear when suspended over a deep "cliff." Fearful reactions including heart rate acceleration, distress, and refusal to cross the deep side of the visual cliff, despite the support provided by clear Perspex typically does not emerge until around 8 months of age, although there is individual variability. These findings show that *the fear* of depth emerges several months after the capacity to *perceive* depth. Campos and his colleagues propose that the decalage is attributable to the fact that the sensation of depth does not initially have any fearful meaning. Once the infant is able to locomote and fall, however, depth becomes a very meaningful clue to danger, and thus begins to elicit fear.

Summary

Social smiling usually begins in the second month, and becomes common and reliable within a few weeks. After an initial period of promiscuous sociability, infants come to reserve their broadest and readiest smiles for familiar people. Five or six months later, several new emotional reactions including stranger anxiety, separation anxiety, the fear of heights, and social attachment all emerge at roughly the same time. Stranger reactions, separation anxiety and social attachment have often been linked in attempted explanations of their emergence, although the contemporaneous emergence of the fear of heights at least raises doubts about these links, as does evidence that stranger and separation anxiety have different origins and times of onset. These issues are explored further in the next section, where the focus is on explanations and interpretations of these milestones of socioemotional development.

❑❑❑

9

Interpretations of Socio-Emotional Milestones

Social Smiling

Psychoanalytic Theory. The pleasurable sensation of need gratification helps to organize perception by making certain stimuli salient. When mother-infant interaction develops favourably, the stimuli that become salient are likely to be features of the mother, especially of her face. At first, this perceptual learning is rather crude: It involves discriminating certain specific aspects of the face a configuration consisting of forehead, eyes, and nose. Once this percept is discriminated from the background stimulation, it becomes a social releaser that elicits the smiling response automatically. Thereafter, any oval stimulus containing the features of eyes can elicit smiles, even if the stimulus does not otherwise look much like a face.

Need and need reduction also help organize memory: The child learns that the appearance of the facial stimuli means that drive reduction is about to take place. Hence, Spitz uses the term "sign gestalt" to refer to the facial features that elicit social smiles.

In terms of this theory, infants do not learn to smile; they learn to notice the features of the face which *automatically* elicit smiling. Of course, if there was no consistent caretaker, or no regular coincidence of certain stimuli and certain drive states, the face gestalt would not be noticed until later, if at all. Early, albeit methodologically weak, studies seemed to support the psychoanalysts' contentions: Ambrose found that social smiles occurred earlier in family reared than institutionally reared infants, while Spitz and Wolf found that social smiling was delayed by cold or hostile mother infant interaction.

The onset of social smiling heralds what Spitz called the stage of the preobject, during which the child does not yet understand the identity of the mother. During this stage, many face-like stimuli elicit smiling, while familiar faces in profile do not. Continued interaction promotes further perceptual refinements until, with time, the recognition of mother becomes so affectively laden that an important new set of cognitive and emotional processes emerge, including evocative (recall) memory, separation anxiety, and stranger anxiety.

The psychoanalytic explanation of the onset of social smiling has a fatal flaw, in that 6-12 week old infants smile not only at faces, but also at a wide range of nonsocial stimuli, such as bells and bull's-eye patterns. The theory cannot explain this, and we must thus doubt the veracity of its explanation regarding the onset of social smiles.

Learning Theory. Learning theorists explain the emergence of social smiling by proposing that the features of the face are associated, through a process of classical conditioning, with the pleasurable state that was brought about by drive reduction or need gratification (resulting from feeding, drinking, keeping warm). Later increases in the frequency of social smiling can be affected by operant contingencies: Parents respond enthusiastically when the infant smiles and thus reward or reinforce smiling. Two crucial studies have demonstrated the classical conditioning and deconditioning of emotions, while others have demonstrated that the frequency of smiling can indeed be increased by reinforcement. Thus, there appears to be some empirical support for this theory's predictions.

Unfortunately, learning theory appears better able to explain the transfer of emotional reactions from one stimulus to another and variations in the frequency of smiling and other emotional expressions than to explain the initial emergence of emotional reactions. In the case of social smiling, for example, we know that contrary to Watson's predictions feeding, holding, or stroking babies does not elicit smiling. Thus there is no known unconditional stimulus that initially and innately elicits smiles, which is crucially important if conditional stimuli (like faces or voices) are later to become effective elicitors of smiles through conditioning. Imitation and observational learning likewise cannot explain the onset of social smiling, because blind babies begin smiling to their parents' voices at the same age as sighted infants. And although the frequency of smiling can be shaped through operant conditioning, it is not plausible to suggest that infants' mouth movements are shaped in successive approximations until recognizable smiles are evident.

Cognitive-Developmental Theory. Drawing on several of Piaget's notions, cognitive developmentalists like Kagan have expanded Hebb's theory to account for the occurrence of smiling as a result of both social and nonsocial stimuli. Kagan proposed that smiling occurs when an environmental event is assimilated to (i.e., fitted into) a central schema. Smiling at faces thus reflects the emergence of recognition memory, and mastery of the task of recognizing, first, faces in general, and later, the mother's face. Smiling at nonsocial stimuli, such as bells and bull's-eyes, is explained by hypothesizing that a new perceptual skill the ability to perceive curvilinear stimuli emerges in the third month.

Before then, infants do not perceive curvilinearity, hence pay little attention to such stimuli, and thus do not smile at them. When the skill first emerges, however, it permits the successful but effortful processing of information, and smiling is thus elicited. After three months, sounds are also processed differently : Earlier, they were only listened to, whereas now they can also be looked at. Practicing this new schema results in smiling.

Cognitive theories such as Kagan's predict inverted U-shaped functions relating the probability of emotional response to the amount of experience infants have had: Smiling should not occur when a schema is first being established nor should it occur when the schema is so well developed that the stimulation is no longer novel. Smiling should be greatest when the stimulus is somewhat novel, and thus somewhat difficult to assimilate to an existing schema. There is, in fact, some empirical support for this hypothesis, albeit in a study concerned with the elicitation of smiles by success in nonsocial tasks, varying in the degree of difficulty. Unlike either the psychoanalytic or learning theory explanations, the quality of the infant-mother interaction is of no consequence to Kagan's theory although the amount of interaction may be important. Emotional developments should occur on schedule, regardless of the child's relationship with its mother, provided that some alternative sources of stimulation are available.

Not all cognitive theorists emphasize discrepancy between stimuli and memory schemas as much as Kagan and Hebb do. Sroufe, for example, has shown that degree of discrepancy can account for the *intensity*, but not for the *hedonic quality*, of an emotional reaction. As a result, the same stimulus can elicit very different emotional responses, depending on the context in which testing takes place. For instance, when mothers wear a mask, 9-12 month old infants will tend to smile or laugh, whereas if it is worn by unfamiliar adults, infants may cringe, turn away, or cry. These findings suggest that infants are capable of much more complex cognitive activities than memory and the perception of discrepancy. Following Bowlby, Sroufe interprets these findings to mean that infants (like adults) are capable of rudimentary cognitive inferences or appraisals, designed to determine whether stimuli are potentially pleasurable or harmful. Kagan, on the other hand, denies the existence of these abilities in the first year of life.

Although the cognitive theory appears to explain the emergence of social smiling more successfully than either the psychoanalytic or learning theory, it can be criticized for underemphasizing biological and biogenetic determinants of behaviour. There is a clear developmental progression from biological, internal elicitation to external environmental elicitation of smiles. Newborns smile quite readily, but only in rapid eye movement states. For a few weeks after birth, they also smile when they are drowsy but not when they are awake. Only after 4-6 weeks of age do infants smile in response to environmental stimulation. This developmental sequence appears to be under maturational control, because premature infants begin to smile at environmental stimuli at the same conceptional age as full-term infants, which is, of course, longer after birth and thus after much more postnatal experience. Twin studies show that monozygotic twins are more alike than dizygotic twins in their tendencies to smile during the first four months of life, suggesting that genetic factors influence individual differences in emotional reactions. Experimental studies confirm the importance of innate determinants of emotional development at least in monkeys. When rhesus monkeys who had been raised in isolation were shown pictures of other monkeys making threats, they responded with aversion or fear, whereas they showed positive reactions when shown pictures of infant monkeys. These reactions did not occur before 8 weeks of age, and could not have been learned or affected by internal schemata given the monkeys' prior isolation. In any event, discrepancy from existing schemata cannot explain why some stimuli elicited positive reactions, while others elicited negative reactions. Thus, at least some complex emotional reactions appear to be elicited innately, despite minimal social experience.

In addition, Kagan's model depends on the development (presumably by maturation) of the capacity to perceive and attend to curvilinear stimuli. There is little independent evidence that such a development takes place. Without this new perceptual skill, Kagan is unable to explain the onset of smiling, not only to faces, but also to bells and bull's-eyes. Sroufe similarly proposes the existence of cognitive mechanisms (appraisal processes) for which there has yet to be independent verification.

Ethological-Adaptational Theory. Evidence concerning maturational and biogenetic influences of emotional development led psychologists to turn toward evolutionary biology, in the form of the ethological-adaptational theory, for insight into the nature of socioemotional development. This theory challenges the notion that emotions are mere expressions of internal states by proposing that emotions are essentially communicative in nature. From this viewpoint, social smiles are viewed as signals indicating that stimulation should be maintained or increased. This view of emotions as communicative signals is supported by findings that interaction is adversely affected when emotional signals deviate from the species–specific norm. Thus, for example, mothers are disappointed by the bland facial expressions of blind babies or babies whose expressions are muted because they have Down's syndrome and infants are upset when adults sit impassively and unresponsively in front of them.

Ethological theorists believe that the emergence of social smiling is maturationally determined, and that the emergence of social smiling marks the beginning of a sensitive period for the development of social attachments a period that is said to end with the emergence of stranger anxiety or wariness. This "explanation" only tells us why infants smile focusing on the hypothetical adaptive value of the behaviour but tells us nothing about *how* by what psychological, cognitive, or neurophysiological mechanism the behaviour is elicited. Thus the ethological-adaptational theory provides a different sort of explanation than do the psychoanalytic, learning, and cognitive theories. The ethological explanation is not open to conclusive verification or refutation but, viewed in the context of mechanisms proposed by the cognitive developmental theorists, may provide the most useful perspective on the development of social smiling.

Stranger Anxiety or Wariness

Psychoanalytic Theory. In terms of Spitz's psychoanalytic theory, the onset of stranger anxiety is predicated on ego development sufficient to permit evocative (i.e., recall) memory. Spitz believed that stranger anxiety results from a rudimentary inference process in which the child compares the stranger to an internal representation of mother. If mother is absent, the child anticipates that she will not be available to meet its needs. As a result, distress occurs. Spitz felt that, as with smiling, the quality of mother—infant interaction affects the expression of stranger anxiety, and as predicted, studies show that negative reactions to strangers are either absent or mild among infants raised in institutions.

One problem with this explanation is that the emergence of stranger anxiety around 6-9 months of age coincides with the emergence of fear to a variety of events or stimuli, such as heights, looming stimuli, masks, and jack-in-the-boxes. It seems unlikely that these emotional changes result from ego development mediated by mother-infant interaction, and thus one wonders whether the explanation of stranger anxiety is correct. Another problem is that the intensity of reactions to strangers appear more related to the amount of experience with strangers than to the quality of infant mother attachment.

Learning Theory. Learning theory is similarly unable to explain the emergence of stranger anxiety. Strangers generally do not hurt or discomfort infants, making a conditioning explanation unlikely. Furthermore, parents are not usually afraid of strangers (especially when the stranger is a relative), so observational learning is clearly not involved. And we are aware of no operant contingencies that can plausibly explain the phenomenon.

Cognitive-Developmental Theory. Cognitive theorists, as in the case of smiling, initially proposed that discrepancies between the features of the stranger and some internal memory or schema explain the occurrence of stranger anxiety, because the child is unable to assimilate the stranger's features to any existing schema. One major problem with this explanation, however, was that infants can visually discriminate between mothers and strangers by 3 months of age but they do not show fear or distress until 4 or 5 months later. Consequently, Kagan, Kearsley, and Zelazo have amended Hebb's basic notions quite substantially, adding the proposition that in the third quarter-year, infants develop the capacity to generate hypotheses, and thereafter actively attempt to understand how the environment operates, instead of merely registering sensory inputs passively. Before this capacity develops, a discrepancy between environmental stimulation and a schema yields interest rather than fear; after 8 months, however, fear or distress results when children attempt to understand environmental events and their hypotheses fail. Kagan thus portrays wariness to unfamiliar stimuli, as well as separation distress, as the predictable results of failures to understand the environment. If the child knew where mother went, when she would return, or what the stranger would do, no negative reactions would result.

Because the quality of mother-infant interaction is not viewed as a determinant of stranger anxiety, Kagan would expect distress or wariness to emerge according to a normative timetable, regardless of differences in prior social experiences. Substantiating this prediction, he has argued that stranger anxiety emerges at about the same time in infants from Israeli kibbutzim, the Kalahari desert, Greek orphanages, Guatemalan Indian groups, and middle-class Massachusetts families.

However, Sroufe believes that discrepancy can account for the intensity, but not the hedonic quality, of emotional reactions to strange people or objects. In his view, hedonic quality is determined by the physical and social context as well as by the child's past experiences. For example, the stranger's approach is more likely to elicit cardiac acceleration and fussing in an unfamiliar setting than in the home. The parents' proximity, as well as their perceived accessibility, also affect reactions to strangers. According to Sroufe, these effects occur because infants have the capacity to *appraise* both stimuli and their contexts in order to determine whether there is reason for fear. Sroufe showed that differences among studies in the amount of wariness observed could be attributed to differences in the contexts in which the observations took place. Thus, when the mother was close by, the infant was familiarized with the stranger, and the stranger did not behave intrusively, stranger distress was often weak, subtle, and intermixed with positive, affiliative behaviours. On the other hand, when a stranger intrusively approached in a bizarre manner, or when the infant had little control over the stranger's behaviour, stranger distress occurred in the majority of infants tested cross-sectionally and was nearly universal when infants were tested longitudinally.

The notion of an appraisal process thus helps to integrate diverse and apparently inexplicable findings, but unfortunately, it is a hypothetical construct that cannot be observed or studied directly. An additional problem with cognitive theories is, as mentioned earlier, that they deny the impact of biogenetic and innate determinants of emotional development. Twin studies showed genetic influences on individual differences in reactions to strangers, while Sackett's study showed that fear emerged on a predictable schedule in rhesus monkeys, despite minimal social experience.

Ethological-Adaptational Theory. These findings are consistent with the assumptions of the ethological-adaptational theory, which holds that stranger anxiety occurs because it is adaptive for infants to avoid potential dangers, just as it is adaptive for them to seek the proximity of protective adults, especially when distressed or frightened. The purpose of stranger distress, from this point of view, is to summon the protective parent. While the other signs of fear mediate flight, ethologists argue that the fear of strangers does not emerge earlier in life than it does because emotions and emotional expressions only emerge when they are biologically adaptive. One explanation for the onset of stranger anxiety at around 8 months, therefore, might be that it coincides with the emergence of independent locomotion (by crawling), which allows infants to wander unsupervised into contact with strange adults. Another is that since fear mediates flight, it should not emerge until flight is possible that is, after locomotion is achieved. Ethological theorists also propose that infants may be biologically prepared to respond to certain cues to danger. Among these are individuals who loom large over infants: strangers who tower over infants are feared more than persons at the infants' level. Likewise, unfamiliar full-size adults are feared more than midgets, and both are feared more than strange children. However, the ethological theory attempts to explain only the whys of stranger anxiety; it does not attempt to explain how, i.e., by what psychological and physiological mechanisms negative stranger reactions are mediated.

Social Cognition. The social-cognitive approach in a sense builds on the notions advanced by Sroufe. Instead of proposing that unfamiliar stimuli are inherently fearful because their behavioural dispositions are unknown, theorists such as Campos propose that such stimuli may be *ambiguous*. In an attempt to resolve the ambiguity, infants look at their mothers' faces for cues about how to respond. If mother looks relaxed and happy, the infant concludes that there is nothing to fear and that the stranger may be fun; if mother looks fearful or unhappy, however, the infant concludes that there is reason to fear or avoid the individual. Consistent with this notion, studies have shown that the mother's expressions have a remarkable effect on the child's willingness to play with novel, attractive toys or to cross the deep side of the visual cliff. This explanation does not of course preclude situations in which the adult's behaviour is sufficiently bizarre, and the context so threatening, that fear is elicited immediately; it deals only with the situation in which ambiguity exists. Campos and Stenberg propose that infants begin to seek information from their parents' emotional expressions by 5 months of age, by which time they clearly seem capable of discriminating among various expressions. Although the social-cognitive approach does not provide a comprehensive account of stranger reactions, the best explanation of stranger wariness is probably provided by an amalgam of the cognitive-developmental, ethological-adaptational, and social-cognitive approaches, each of which seeks to explain different aspects of the phenomenon.

Separation Anxiety

Psychoanalytic Theory. Each of the major theories proposes an explanation of separation anxiety very similar to its explanation of stranger anxiety. In the case of psychoanalytic theory, Spitz proposed that stranger anxiety actually occurred because the infant feared separation from its mother. In his view, separation anxiety first becomes possible when evocative memory develops between 6 and 8 months of age; this allows the infant to retrieve an image of mother in her absence. Prior to this time, the infant could recognize mother, but could not recall her image in her absence. Out of sight was out of mind. The ability to remember mother, even in her absence, permits the baby to feel threatened by her absence, and this threat is signaled by anxiety. The belief that recall memory is available by 6-8 months contradicted Piaget's belief that this is not possible until the second year, but Spitz argued that there was a decalage attributable to the organizing effect of affect on cognitive growth. Specifically, he proposed that the ability to understand mother's permanence precedes the ability to understand the permanence of objects, because mother is more affectively salient. This crucial assumption has not been empirically supported, however. Jackson, Campos, and Fischer found that when hide-and-search tasks are made comparable, infants show an equivalent appreciation of object and person permanence and search in very similar ways for both their mothers and toys. This constitutes a fatal flaw in the psychoanalytic explanations of separation anxiety and stranger anxiety.

Learning Theory. Learning theorists explain separation anxiety by suggesting that it represents the withdrawal of a source of both positive gratification and contingent responding. This explanation can satisfactorily explain the onset of distress when the separation occurs, but it cannot explain the later emergence of a qualitatively different reaction, despair, and the subsequent emergence of detachment. Qualitative changes in the reaction to prolonged separation suggest that something more complex occurs than is proposed by learning theorists.

Cognitive-Developmental Theorists. To theorists like Kagan, separation produces a discrepancy from the familiar schema in which mother is present. The child thus generates hypotheses in an attempt to explain what happened to mother. Not knowing what happened to her, or when she will return, the child's hypotheses fail and distress results. Separation protest does not occur before 6-8 months because younger infants are not capable of generating hypotheses. The viability of this explanation thus depends on the assumption that the capacity to demonstrate hypotheses emerges around 6-8 months of age. No evidence of this sort has yet been presented.

Ethological-Adaptational Theory. Theorists such as Bowlby perceive separation distress as a signal by the infant designed to summon the absent parent back into proximity. Separation protest is thus viewed as one of several attachment behaviours that promote proximity between infants and attachment figures. Some attachment behaviours, like separation protest, bring about proximity only when the infant's signal successfully elicits an approach by the adult. Others, like locomotor approach, depend on the infant's behaviour alone. Attachment behaviours, like separation protest, are said to emerge around 7-8 months of age because this is the age at which infants first appreciate person permanence, and thus can be said to have established social relationships. This assumption is the same as that made by Spitz, and is similarly unsupported by the empirical evidence. Thus, while the ethological-adaptational theory may have been correct in identifying the adaptive purpose of separation protest, Bowlby was unsuccessful in his attempt to explain the emergence of separation protest at 6-8 months of age. A better explanation, consistent with the ethological perspective, might be that separation protest does not emerge until the onset of locomotor capacities makes it possible for the child to wander off, and thus find itself separated from an attachment figure.

Social Cognition. Proponents of a social-cognitive approach have not attempted to explain the onset of separation protest. However, researchers have used this perspective to help understand individual differences in infants' behaviour upon reunion after brief separations.

Social Attachment

There is considerable overlap between the predictions and assumptions regarding social attachment and those concerning separation anxiety, stranger anxiety, and (to a lesser extent) social smiling. This is because some theorists view social attachment simply as a summary term referring to all discriminating social behaviours, while others believe that such behaviours mediate and manifest an underlying social bond, which continues to exist even at times when no attachment behaviours are occurring. To psychoanalysts, for example, the onset of separation and stranger anxiety is determined by ego development bringing about the capacity for evocative memory. Separation and stranger anxiety are viewed simply as behavioural manifestations of a change in the infant's inner socioemotional world.

Psychoanalytic Theory. Psychoanalytic theorists have, since the time of Freud, emphasized the crucial importance of the infant-mother relationship, which Freud described as "unique, without parallel, established unalterably for the whole lifetime as the prototype of all later love relations". This emphasis derived from the assumption that the most important interactions between parents and young infants were those around feeding. Bonds were deemed most likely to form to those who satisfied the infant's hunger, on the grounds that drive reduction was gratifying and that bonds were thus formed to those consistently responsible for this gratification.

Learning Theory. The psychoanalysts' secondary drive interpretation was adopted nearly intact by learning theorists like Hull, who attempted a reinterpretation in learning terms of central psychoanalytic mechanisms and processes. Later learning theorists also emphasized the association between features of the caretaker and the gratification implicit in feeding. In the most popular recent interpretations of early attachment in the context of learning theory, Gewirtz and Bijou and Baer have provided operant conditioning models in which the mother becomes a discriminant reinforcer. One major difference between learning theorists and the psychoanalysts is that learning theorists eschew discussion of hypothetical structures like the ego, and deny the existence of emotional bonds independent of observable behaviours.

Both the psychoanalytic and learning theory explanations were fatally compromised by research showing that feeding does not play a crucial role in attachment. In one famous study, Harlow and Zimmerman showed that infant monkeys sought comfort from, and preferred to cling to, a terrycloth mother surrogate rather than a wire surrogate, which fed them. These studies, coupled with the general fall from favour of drive reduction theories, led developmental psychologists to abandon both psychoanalytic and learning theory accounts of social attachment, and paved the way for Bowlby's new ethological-adaptational theory. Gewirtz's theory also cannot explain why abused infants cling to, rather than flee, abusive parents; why infants first protest and then grieve over the loss of parents; and why infants use attachment figures as "secure bases" from which to explore. All of these behaviour patterns are consistent with the ethological-adaptational model, which links the formation of attachments to the infants' need for protection from more powerful and competent adults.

Ethological-Adaptational Theory. Like the psychoanalysts, Bowlby believed that separation anxiety reflected the establishment of a bond between infant and mother. However, he attempted to replace the secondary drive explanation, implicit in psychoanalytic theory, with an explanation that was more consistent with the postulates of contemporary biology. He believed that infants were equipped with a repertoire of behaviours that served to promote proximity and contact with adults and were thus of survival value. In young infants, the proximity-promoting behaviours initially consisted of signals (such as smiles and cries) that were effective in achieving proximity or contact only when they elicited the responses with which adults were preprogrammed to respond. The fact that proximity depended on the association of infant behaviours and complementary adult responses is important because attachments apparently form to those individuals who are consistently available and respond in appropriate fashion to the infant's signals.

Bowlby proposed that there were several discrete stages in the development of attachment. Initially, the child is promiscuously sociable, not caring who responds to its proximity-promoting signals (0-6 weeks). Once it achieves the capcity to distinguish among individuals, it begins to demonstrate preferences, which become increasingly marked over the ensuing months. However, attachments are not said to form until the appreciation of person permanence, around 7-8 months of age, makes it possible for the child to remain aware of the adult's existence even when he/she is not audible or visible. At this point, an attachment bond is said to exist. The bond can be identified by seeing to whom the infant directs its proximity-promoting signals, but (and this is a crucial assumption) these behaviours only mediate the bond they are not equivalent to the bond. Among the attachment behaviours are separation protest, locomotor approach, clinging, asking to be held, staying close, directed crying, and use of the adult as a "secure base" from which to explore.

Cognitive-Developmental Theory. Cognitive theorists like Kagan do not attempt to explain the development of attachment bonds. They believe that the bond is really a composite of behavioural changes that can be attributed to emergent cognitive capacities. Others, such as Sroufe, accept Bowlby's explanation of the development of attachment. However, Sroufe has drawn upon cognitive development to explain the appraisal process by which infants determine how much proximity/contact they need (the set goal) given the existing circumstances and their locomotor capacities, and compare that with the degree of proximity/contact currently being enjoyed. Any discrepancy between present status and the set goal sets in motion behaviours designed to restore the balance.

Social Cognition. Finally, social cognitive theorists focus not on the formation of social bonds, but on the way in which differences in parental behavioural styles presage the development of distinctive social expectations of those adults' future behaviour. The latter issues is discussed further in the section on individual differences.

Fear of Heights

The psychoanalysts and learning theorists have not attempted to explain the emergence of the fear of heights. The cognitive-developmental and ethological adaptational theorists offer explanations one focused on proximal mechanisms and one on the adaptive value of the fear. The proponents of a social-cognitive approach have also considered ways in which the intensity of fear can be modulated.

Cognitive-Developmental Theory. Theorists such as Kagan propose that the fear of heights can be explained in the same way as the fear of strangers. In each case, there is a discrepancy between the current percept and the child's mental schemata, which are based on past experiences. Discrepancy is perceived by 2-3 months, but it elicits interest rather than distress prior to the emergence, around 8 months of age, of the capacity to generate hypotheses. The failure of these hypotheses is said to underlie the emergence of frank distress. As before, a crucial problem with this explanation is the lack of independent evidence that the capacity to generate hypotheses indeed emerges at this time.

Ethological-Adaptational Theory. From this point of view, the fear of heights is an adaptive emotion that mediates avoidance of heights and, in so doing, protects the infant from the danger of falling. Theorists such as Izard believe that emotions emerge when they are adaptive, and thus it is not surprising that the fear of heights emerges when the child acquires the ability to locomote independently (by crawling) and is thus exposed for the first time to the danger of falling. Consistent with this, Campos and his colleagues have shown that the fear of heights predictably emerges shortly after the acquisition of the ability to locomote independently. Age is not the critical variable, because the emergence of fear can be accelerated by giving infants the opportunity for independent locomotion using walkers before they are able to crawl. It is not yet clear, however, whether the experience of falling is also crucial.

Social Cognition. Campos and his colleagues have also shown that the magnitude of fear can be manipulated by varying the emotional cues provided by the child's mother in ambiguous situations. For example, when the drop-off is small (e.g., one foot on the visual cliff), the child is uncertain whether the depth is sufficient to elicit fear, and looks to its mother's face for disambiguating information. If mother smiles and talks in a positive tone, infants are likely to cross the deep cliff to mother, whereas if mother produces a fear face and talks in a negative or fearful tone, infants are very unlikely to cross the same cliff. Of course, if there was no depth or the cliff was clearly very deep, the mother's cues would be less influential because there would be little ambiguity in the child's mind, and thus little reason to seek disambiguating information.

Summary

Learning theory does a poor job of explaining the discrete and abrupt emergence of emotional milestones, while the psychoanalytic theory is flawed by the unwarranted linking of stranger and separation anxiety, and by the recourse to unobservable and unverifiable aspects of ego development. Kagan's cognitive-developmental theory has uncertain status until it is possible to demonstrate that the ability to generate hypotheses indeed emerges around 8 months of age; it also has to acknowledge the importance of biogenetic factors as determinants of emotional development. Sroufe's cognitive developmental theory is more successful in explaining both the intensity and hedonic quality of emotional reactions, and is most readily integrated with Bowlby's ethological-adaptational theory. The ethological-adaptational theory has been extremely influential because it has provided a way of explaining why we should expect to see certain emotions developing, and why they should emerge when they do. However, only in the case of social attachments have theorists like Bowlby attempted to explain the proximal mechanisms involved.

In part because of the lack of alternatives, most researchers and theorists today accept Bowlby's theory as the most useful, and agree that a major change in the nature of the infant's social world takes place around 6-8 months of age although (ironically) the empirical evidence shows that this change cannot be attributed to the emergence of person permanence. Bowlby's emphasis on the survival functions of infant behaviour has been tremendously valuable, because it has allowed researchers to perceive organization and purpose in infant behaviour that formerly appeared merely disorganized and incompetent. Further, his suggestion that bonds form as a result of consistent and appropriate adult responses to proximity-promoting behaviours provides a plausible and testable explanation of the way in which adult-child interaction affects the formation of infant-adult attachments. On the other hand, Bowlby's belief that infants are limited to forming one attachment initially has been disproved by evidence that infants generally form attachments to both parents at the same time even though (consistent with Bowlby's emphasis) most seem to establish preferential relationships with their primary caretakers. These preferences are evident in times of stress, when the infants' need for proximity to trusted protective adults is at its greatest. Most researchers agree that the *amount* of interaction is not critical to the formation of attachments or even to the establishment of preferences; the *quality* of interaction (as manifest by the adult's characteristic degree of responsiveness to the infant's signals) is more important. In the case of traditional fathers who spend relatively little time interacting with their infants, a propensity for exciting playful stimulation seems to increase the salience of their interactions and permit infants to establish attachment relationships to them.

Individual Differences in Socio-emotional Development

The study of individual differences has been the major concern of theorists and researchers in the last decade, with focus being placed on the quality or security of infant-adult attachment. Coherence in this area has been facilitated greatly by the availability of a procedure the Strange Situation by which security of attachment can be assessed; almost all recent research on this topic has involved this procedure. As far as emotional development is concerned, dimensions of expressiveness or emotionality, as well as sociability or friendliness, have been of paramount concern, but there has been less agreement about how these are to be defined, much less studied. Consequently, the literature appears non-programmematic and disjointed.

Social Development

Both the psychoanalytic and (implicitly) learning theory approaches to the study of social development deal with individual differences in socioemotional development, to the extent that variations in the quality of mother-infant interaction may retard development. However, most of the relevant, empirical work undertaken by psychoanalytic theorists involved comparing children raised in home settings with those raised in institutions such as orphanages, where care by a succession of shift nurses replaced normal mother-infant interaction. Variations within the normal range have been explored by psychoanalysts only in the context of case reports. Learning theorists, by contrast, seemed able to explain the effects of a wide variety of mother-child interaction patterns, until it was demonstrated that individual differences, as assessed by discrete behavioural measures, were highly unstable even over short periods of time. Since the learning theorists refused to acknowledge constructs other than those at the discrete behavioural level, these findings undercut the theory's ability to describe or explain stable individual differences. Cognitive theorists like Kagan, meanwhile, had placed such great stress on normative maturational events that there was no room to accommodate individual differences: Indeed, several reports focused on the absence of developmental variation despite vast differences in rearing environments.

By contrast, the ethological-adaptational theorists seem to have been most successful in their efforts to explore the origins, characteristics, and consequences of individual differences in infant-parent attachment. Perhaps the major reason for the apparent success of these theorists is their focus, not on discrete behaviours, but on the patterned organization of behaviour.

The ethological-adaptational theorists believe that infants are born with a repertoire of proximity-promoting signals to which adults are predisposed to respond. The formation of attachments depends on the continued presence and responsiveness of specific adults during the first 6 months or so of life. Adults differ in their responsiveness to infants, however, and these differences in responsiveness are viewed as the antecedents of individual differences in the later quality of infant-adult attachments.

According to theorists such as Ainsworth, these individual differences can best be assessed by observing the effect of stress on the infant's behaviour, because stress should increase the infant's desire for proximity to and/or contact with the protective parent or attachment figure, thus leading to the intensification of the "attachment behaviour system" that controls a variety of behaviours (as diverse as crying, approaching, and clinging) that have the common function of helping infants attain or maintain proximity/contact. Thus, as the stress increases, infants should reduce their exploration and affiliation (for example, with strangers) and increasingly organise their behaviour around their parents. Specifically, they should evince distress when separated from their parents, attempt to search for them, and greet them with bids for renewed interaction, either in the form of proximity/contact or in the form of distance interaction.

Operationally, individual differences in response to stress are usually assessed using a procedure the Strange Situation developed by Ainsworth and Wittig. The procedure is designed to subject 10-24-month-old infants to gradually increasing amounts of stress, induced by the strange setting, the entrance of a strange female, and two brief separations from the parent.

Ainsworth's research, and that of other researchers in this tradition, has repeatedly shown that when infants and parents are observed in the Strange Situation, about 65-75% behave in the pattern described above, which is termed the secure (or B) pattern because the infant seems to gain security and comfort from the parent to whom it turns in times of stress or alarm. The remainder display one of two types of reactions. Typically, 20-25% behave in an avoidant (A) fashion, turning away from, rather than toward the adult, especially upon reunion, when one would expect proximity-seeking behaviours to be at their most intense. Another group, the resistant, or C, group comprising 10-15% of most samples, consists of infants who are unable to use the adult as a base for exploration even in the preseparation episodes. These infants behave in an ambivalent fashion upon reunion both seeking contact and angrily rejecting it when offered. These patterns of behaviour seem to be characteristic of specific relationships, because infants may behave differently with their mothers and fathers. The patterns are not ephemeral, however; infants who are seen in the Strange Situation more than once with the same adult tend to behave similarly in each observation, provided that no major changes in family circumstances or caretaking arrangements take place between the two assessments. The fact that changes in family circumstances affect behaviour in the Strange Situation supports the assumption that this behaviour is determined by prior patterns of infant-parent interaction, as does evidence that abused infants are more likely to develop insecure attachments to their abusive mothers.

All episodes are usually three minutes long, but episodes 3, 5, and 6 can be curtailed if the infant is too distressed, and episodes 4 and 7 are sometimes extended.

Further evidence in support of this assumption was gathered by Ainsworth and her colleagues in a small longitudinal study. Infants who behaved in the normative or secure pattern in the Strange Situation had mothers who responded promptly and appropriately to the infants' signals and needs when observed at home. Those who behaved avoidantly or resistantly had less sensitively responsive mothers. One difference between these two groups was that the mothers of avoidant infants were conspicuously rejecting and, since they found physical contact distasteful, their attempts to soothe were often abrupt. The behaviour of the mothers of resistant infants was inconsistent and unpredictable.

Table 9.1. The Strange Situation

Episode	Persons Present	Change
1	Parent, Infant	Enter room
2	Parent, Infant, Stranger	Strange adult joins the dyad
3	Infant, Stranger	Parent leaves
4	Parent, Infant	Parent returns
		Stranger leaves
5	Infant	Parent leaves
6	Infant, Stranger	Stranger returns
7	Parent, Infant	Parent returns
		Stranger leaves

Although these findings are frequently considered definitive, it is important to note that they were obtained in a small exploratory study using a methodology that would be inappropriate for hypothesis testing. The findings have not been independently replicated despite several attempts to verify or replicate them. At this point, findings only show clearly that low-quality maternal care is associated with the development of insecure attachments. Considerably more research is needed on the antecedents of security of attachment.

Drawing upon Ainsworth findings, nevertheless, Lamb has attempted to explain the relationship between security of attachment and prior patterns of infant-adult interaction by proposing that behaviour in the Strange Situation reflects the infants' expectations about the adult's likely behaviour based on the infants' past experiences with that adult. Thus securely attached infants have come to count on or trust the adult, who has in the past responded promptly and appropriately to the infant's signals or needs. By contrast, some infants behave avoidantly because, on the basis of their past experiences, they expect rebuffs rather than comfort in the Strange Situation. To avoid rebuffs, they turn away from the person whose responses have tended to be aversive in the past. Resistant infants do not know what to expect of adults whose behaviour has been so unreliable and unpredictable in the past. This inability to predict the adults' behaviour may underlie the ambivalent and confused behaviour of resistant infants in the Strange Situation. In the absence of reliable information about the antecedents of attachment security, these interpretations are, of course, highly speculative.

Individual differences in Strange Situation behaviour appear to predict the infants' future behaviour, and this has enhanced the popularity of the Strange Situation. Researchers have shown that securely attached infants are more friendly and sociable with unfamiliar peers and adults, both contemporaneously and as much as several years after assessment in the Strange Situation, than are infants who were insecurely attached.

Other studies suggest that securely attached infants are more persistent and resourceful in challenging tasks, at least through 5 years of age. However, predictions over long periods of time are only significant when there is stability in security of attachment, family circumstances, and/or caretaking arrangements. Perhaps, therefore, the apparent "predictive validity" simply involves relationships between the outcome measures and characteristics of the contemporaneous (rather than former) attachment relationship. Consequently, it is not clear just how important an effect security of attachment has on later development.

Emotional Development

Individual differences in emotional development have received little attention other than in the late 1940s and early 1950s, and in the last several years. Interest in the 1940s and 1950s was prompted by evidence concerning the effects of institutionalization on social and emotional development. Children who had grown up in institutions frequently seemed to display a listless, affectless demeanor, showed no interest in social interaction, and failed to display appropriate emotions in situations that should have elicited either pleasure or distress.

Bowlby attributed this "affectionless personality" to a history of "maternal deprivation," and his interpretation played a major role in prompting development of the ethological-adaptational theory. The studies from this era have been soundly criticized, however, mainly for their reliance on retrospective research strategies. In the most thorough critique, Rutter has shown that long-term effects on personality are not inevitable; they depend on the child's constitutional vulnerability or invulnerability, as well as on the occurrence of other traumatic experiences before or after parent-child separation. This casts doubt on the ballistic view of social and emotional development typically held by psychoanalysts.

In the last few years, researchers have focused on variations in the quality of infant-mother relationships, rather than on the effects of separation. Interest in the origins of individual differences in emotional development was rekindled by evidence that (1) there were patterns of emotional expression that had similar communicative meanings around the world; (2) emotional expressions were "appropriately" displayed by young infants in affect-eliciting contexts. Once researchers knew that they could code and interpret infant expressions, reliable and valid research became possible and a variety of experiential influences on emotionality have since been studied. Researchers such as Gaensbauer, for example, have compared the emotional expressions of abused and neglected infants with those who have no history of abuse or neglect. Gaensbauer and his colleagues showed that abused infants evinced a flattening of emotional expressiveness reminiscent of the emotional blunting observed in institutionalized infants. In a detailed case study, Stem showed that intrusive overstimulation led an infant to become avoidant of eye-contact with its mother, whereas mothers who were sensitive to their infants' readiness for stimulation had infants who were more sociable and expressive.

Another strategy has involved comparing infants who behaved differently in the Strange Situation, on the assumption that differences in Strange Situation behaviour are consequences of differences in the quality of infant-mother interaction. Thus Thompson and Lamb found that securely attached infants were more emotionally expressive in the Strange Situation than either avoidant or resistant infants were. They speculated that these differences could be attributed to differences in the patterns of early interaction, suggesting that compared with less sensitive mothers, sensitively responsive mothers were more likely to (1) provide emotionally arousing stimuli at times when their infants were best able to appreciate them; (2) reinforce and encourage emotional displays; (3) be more sensitive to subtle variations in infant expressions. Those infants who were highly expressive facially were also most expressive vocally, suggesting that a general cross-modal dimension of expressiveness exists. This dimension is probably not of direct temperamental origin, because there are few relationships between parental reports of infant temperament and measures of facial or vocal expressiveness.

Another aspect of emotional expressiveness is "sociability", the infant's social attractiveness, friendliness, and willingness to respond positively to social bids by others. Individual differences in sociability appear to be consistent across contexts and moderately stable over a period of several months, provided there is stability in the security of attachment. This suggests that individual differences in sociability are affected by prior social experiences. However, although there is a modest relationship between security of attachment and sociability with unfamiliar adults and peers, there is no significant relationship between sociability and amount of experience with adults, maternal employment or the amount of non-maternal care. Infants appear to be modestly more sociable when their fathers are highly involved in child care.

Whereas the experiential determinants of individual differences in sociability remain unknown, there is mounting evidence of biogenetic influences. The fact that the similarities between monozygotic twins pairs are greater than those between dizygotic twins suggests that sociability is at least somewhat heritable.

Research on the heritability of sociability is related to research on temperament, typically defined as a constitutionally determined behavioural style which is somewhat stable over time. Most studies have focused on some or all of the nine dimensions described by Thomas, Chess, Birch, Hertzig and Korn in their New York Longitudinal Study: rhythm, persistence, threshold, approach, adaptability, activity, intensity, mood, and distractability. Studies using both objective measures as well as more subjective parental reports suggest that there is substantial heritability in at least some dimensions of temperament. Currently, the most exciting research regarding temperament has to do with the relationship between objective indices and parental reports, the heritability of temperament and the way in which child and parent characteristics combine to affect the child's development.

Summary

Theorists concerned with the origins of individual differences in social and emotional behaviour have generally assumed that these differences are determined by differences in the child's early social experiences. Major focus has fallen on the concept, parental sensitivity, which is rather loosely defined and operationalized. This has made it difficult to identify which aspects of parental behaviour are especially important, and whether the effects on security of attachment are influenced by the same aspects of parental behaviour as emotional expressiveness or sociability. More recently, researchers have recognised that at least some aspects of socioemotional development are affected by heredity. Future work is likely to focus on the ways in which inherent differences interact with aspects of the child's environment to determine individual differences.

On the basis of evidence now available, it seems that the understanding of socioemotional development, and of infancy in general, is considerably advanced by the perspective of evolutionary biology, which has provided a way of making sense of infant behaviour simply by proposing that we consider the adaptive significance and function of infant behaviour. This has provided answers to questions about why social smiling, stranger anxiety, separation anxiety, social attachment, and the fear of heights occur at all, and why they emerge when they do. This perspective, however, tells us little about the mechanisms whereby these phenomena are mediated, and nothing about the way in which individual differences in social and emotional development are to be explained. With respect to the hows of development, the most useful answers have come from the cognitive-developmental theorists, especially those like

Sroufe who have attempted to make their propositions consistent with the ethological-adaptational theory. Biogenetic approaches emphasizing heritability, the analysis of social interaction, and social-cognitive perspectives seem most likely to contribute to our understanding of individual differences.

❑❑❑

Bibliography

Allison, R. with Schwarz, T. (1999). *Minds in many pieces: Revealing the Spiritual Side of Multiple Personality Disorder*. Los Osos, CA: CIE Publishing.

Arnold, E.C. (1978). Role-playing helps detect fact-finding gaps. *Community College Journalist, 7*, 1. 8-10.

Avens, R. (1980). *Imagination is Reality: Western nirvana in Jung, Hillman, Barfield & Cassirer*. Dallas, TX. Spring.

Bateson, G., Jackson, D.D., Haley, J. & Weakland, J.H. (1956). Toward a theory of schizophrenia. *Behavioral Science, 1*, 251-64.

Beaton, D. I. (1987). *The Impact of Residential Treatment on Interpersonal and Intrapsychic Dimensions of Schizophrenia* [CD-ROM]. Abstract from: Dissertation Abstracts International, Vol. 48-08B.

Campbell, J. (1968/1949). *The Hero with a Thousand Faces*. Princeton, NJ: Princeton University Press.

Campbell, J., and Oakes, M. (1969). *Where the two came to their Father: A Navaho war ceremonial*. Princeton, NJ: Princeton University Press.

Davis, G.A. & Houtman, S.E. (1968). *Thinking Creatively: A Guide to Training Imagination*. Madison: University of Wisconsin.

Dokter, D. (1998) (Ed.). *Arts Therapists, Refugees and Migrants: Reaching across Borders*. London: Jessica Kingsley

Edinger, E.F. (1972). *Ego & Archetype: Individuation and the Religious Function of the Psyche*. Boston: Shambhala.

Edinger, E.F. (1991). *Anatomy of the Psyche: Alchemical Symbolism in Psychotherapy.* La Salle, IL: Open Court. (Original work published 1985)

Edinger, E.F. (1996). *The New God Image: A Study of Jung's Key Letters Concerning the Evolution of the Western God-image.* Wilmette, IL: Chiron.

Fairbairn, W.R.D. (1940). Schizoid factors in the personality. *Psychoanalytic Studies of the Personality* 3-27. London: Routledge and Kegan Paul.

Fischer, K.W., Shaver, P.R., & Carnochan, P. (1990). *How Emotions Develop and How They Organize Development. Cognition & Emotion, 4.* 81-127.

Gardner, H. (1983). *Frames of Mind: The Theory of Multiple Intelligences.* United States: Basic Books.

Gilligan, C. (1993). *In a Differer ' Voice: Psychological Theory and Women's Development.* Cambridge: Harvard University Press.

Harrell, M.D. (1987). *Women without Worlds: Splitting in the Feminine Psyche* [CD-ROM]. Abstract from: Dissertation Abstracts International, Vol. 48-08B.

Hartmann, H. (1939). *Ego Psychology and the Problem of Adaptation.* New York: International University Press.

Jacobi, J. (1959). *Complex, Archetype, Symbol in the Psychology of C.G. Jung.* (R. Manheim, trans.) Princeton, NJ: Princeton University Press.

Kalsched, D. (1996). *The Inner World of Trauma: Archetypal Defense of the Personal Spirit.* London: Routledge.

Kast, V. (1993). *Imagination as Space of Freedom: Dialogue Between the Ego and the Unconscious.* (A. Hollo, Trans.). New York: Fromm International.

Layard, J. (1975). *A Cceltic Quest: Sexuality and Soul in Individuation. A Depth-psychology Study of the Mabinogion Legend of Culhwch and Olwen.* Zurich: Spring.

Lenhart, D.S. (1988). *The children of Ganymede: An Investigation into the Symbolic Language of Gay Men through the Use of Sandplay Therapy* [CD-ROM]. Abstract from: Dissertation Abstracts International, Vol. 50-04B.

Mahler, M.S., Pine, F. & Bergman, A. (1975). *The Psychological Birth of the Human Infant: Symbiosis and Individuation.* New York: Basic Books, Inc.

Meade, M. (1993). *Men and the Water of Life: Initiation and the Tempering of Men.* New York: HarperSan Francisco.

Meador, B.D.S. (1994). *Uncursing the Dark: Treasures from the Underworld.* Wilmette, ILL: Chiron Publications.

Neumann, E. (1971). *The Origins and History of Consciousness* (R.F.C. Hull, Trans.). Princeton, NJ: Princeton University Press.

Neumann, E. (1972). *The Great Mother: An Analysis of the Archetype* (R. Manheim, Trans.). Princeton, NJ: Princeton University Press. (Original work published 1955)

Neumann, E. (1972). *The Great Mother: An Analysis of the Archetype.* (R. Manheim, Trans.). (Original work published 1955)

Ogden, T.H. (1982). *Projective Identification and Psychotherapeutic Technique.* New York: Jason Aronson.

Otto, R. (1950). *The Idea of the Holy: An Inquiry into the Non-rational Factor in the Idea of the Divine and its Relation to the Rational* (J.W. Harvey, Trans., 2nd ed.). London: Oxford University Press.

Perry, B.D. (2001). The neuroarcheology of childhood maltreatment: The neurodevelopmetnal costs of adverse childhood events. *The Cost of Maltreatment: Who Pays? We all do,* 15-37. (K. Franey, R. Geffner & R. Falconer, Eds.) San Diego, CA: Family Violence and Sexual Assault Institute.

Perry, B.D. (2002). Childhood experience and the expression of genetic potential: What childhood neglect tells us about nature and nurture. *Brain and Mind, 3,* 79-100.

Raff, J. (2000). *Jung and The Alchemical Imagination.* York Beach, ME: Nicolas-Hays.

Randour, M. (Ed.). (1993). *Exploring Sacred Landscapes: Religious and Spiritual Experiences in Psychotherapy.* New York: Columbia University Press.

Samuels, A. (Ed.), (1985). *The Father: Contemporary Jungian Perspectives.* New York: New York University Press.

Sandner, D., Wong, S. (1997). *The Sacred Heritage: The Influence of Shamanism on Analytical Psychology.* NY: Routledge.

Stone, H. & Winkelman (1986). *Voice Dialogue: A Tool for Transformation.* Marina Del Rey: De Vorse and Company

Stroul, B., & Friedman, R.M. (1986). *A System of Care for Children and Adolescents with Severe Emotional Disturbances.* xxiv. Washington, D.C.: Georgetown University Child Development Center, National Technical Assistance Center for Children's Mental Health.

Sutton-Smith, B. (2002). Recapitulation redressed. Roopnarine, I. (Ed.), *Conceptual Social-cognitive, and Contexual Issues in the Fields of Play,* Play & Culture Studies, Vol. 4. Westport, CT: Ablex.

Turner, V. (1974). Dramas, Fields, and Metaphors: Symbolic Action in Human Society. Ithaca, NY: Cornell University Press.

von Franz, M.-L. (1980). *Projection and Re-collection in Jungian Psychology: Reflections of the Soul.* London: Open Court.

Winnicott, D.W. (1992). Transitional objects and transitional phenomena. (Originally published 1951). *Through Paediatrics to Psycho-Analysis: Collected Papers,* pp.229-242.

Young-Eisendrath, P., and Dawson, T. (1997). *The Cambridge Companion to Jung.* Cambridge, UK: Cambridge University Press.

Index

Other Books on

EDUCATION

1.	Educational Thought and Practice (New)	195/-
2.	Guidance and Counselling : A Manual (New)	175/-
3.	School Organization and Administration (New)	195/-
4.	Developmental Psychology (New)	195/-
5.	Social Work : Theory and Practice (New)	225/-
6.	History of Ancient India (New)	395/-
7.	Select World Constitutions (New)	395/-
8.	Modern Education for New Generation (New)	175/-
9.	Advanced Educational Technology (New)	175/-
10.	Comparative Education (New)	175/-
11.	Introduction to Educational Research (New)	175/-
12.	Computer Education (New)	175/-
13.	Teaching of Chemistry (New)	175/-
14.	Teaching of Physics (New)	175/-
15.	Handbook of Journalism & Mass Media (New)	225/-
16.	Advanced Educational Psychology	175/-
17.	Educational Administration & Origanisation Management	175/-
18.	Social Psychology	225/-
19.	Teaching of Commerce	175/-
20.	Educational Development & Technology	175/-
21.	Disaster Management	175/-
22.	Information Technology	175/-
23.	Human Resource Development	175/-
24.	Mass Media Communication	225/-
25.	Adult Education	175/-
26.	General Psychology	175/-
27.	Distance Education in India	175/-
28.	Teacher Education	175/-
29.	Educational Philosophy	175/-
30.	Science Teaching in Schools	150/-
31.	Indian Polity (Revised Edition)	295/-
32.	New Comparative Government (Revised Edition)	295/-
	Advanced (Study in the History of Modern India (PB)	
33.	(Volume-1: 1707-1813)	225/-
34.	(Volume-2: 1813-1920)	325/-
35.	(Volume-3: 1920-1947)	175/-

36. Handbook of Nutrition & Dietetics (New) 250/-
37. Development of Education in India 175/-
38. A Textbook of Environmental Studies 175/-
39. Teaching of History 175/-
40. Administrative Thinkers .175/-
41. Research Methodology 175/-
42. Curriculum Development 195/-
43. Teaching of Science 175/-
44. Teaching of Mathematics 175/-
45. Principles of Educational &Vocational Guidance 175/-
46. Child Psychology 175/-
47. Abnormal Psychology 175/-
48. Indian Education in Emerging Society 175/-
49. Human Resource Management 160/-
50. Higher Education and Global Challenges 175/-
51. Teaching of Geography 150/-
52. Teaching of Social Studies 150/-
53. Teaching of English 175/-
54. Principles of Office Management (Revised Edition) 250/-
55. Education for All: The Indian Saga 175/-
56. Value Education in Global Perspective 175/-
57. Teacher Training 175/-
58. Public Administration 150/-
59. Public Relations and Integrated Communications 195/-
60. Educational Psychology 175/-
61. Introduction to Educational Technology 175/-
62. Textbook of Food and Nutrition 150/-